In this book we will introduce you to a number of easy-to-apply, nonmedical lifestyle improvements that you can start using right away, this very day, to gain control of your blood pressure. If your blood pressure is currently borderline high, and if you haven't yet gone on medication, you may find that by faithfully following the regimens laid out in this book, your problem will resolve itself on its own. If, on the other hand, you're already taking hypertensive medications, these techniques will serve as a powerful supplement to conventional medical treatments, and may even allow you to take smaller doses.

# CONTROLLING HIGH BLOOD PRESSURE THE NATURAL WAY

David L. Carroll
with
Wahida Karmally, M.S.

BALLANTINE BOOKS • NEW YORK

A Ballantine Book
Published by The Ballantine Publishing Group
Copyright © 2000 by David L. Carroll

www.randomhouse.com/BB/

Library of Congress Catalog Card Number: 99-091090

ISBN 0-345-43146-4

Manufactured in the United States of America

First Edition: January 2000

OPM  15  14  13  12  11  10  9  8  7

# Contents

# PART I

## All about High Blood Pressure

# 1

## What This Book Will Do for You

### High Blood Pressure: How Much Should It Worry You?

If you have hypertension—high blood pressure—and if you've discussed this matter with a knowledgeable health care professional, probably the first thing you were told is that this all-too-common disorder is known as the silent killer.

Silent? Killer?

Why?

Because in all but the most serious cases high blood pressure produces no conspicuous symptoms and causes no measurable distress. Indeed, hypertension can work its mischief in a person for years, decades even, without detection. People can go about their daily activities, working, playing, sleeping, eating, feeling healthy and trim the entire time, and never once suspect that a problem lurks.

Until one day it's too late.

Now, all this is true; there is no doubt about it. Elevated blood pressure does its dirty work in the dark, leaving no trace until the damage is done.

At the same time, there is nothing really "silent" about hypertension if you know what to look for.

And the ailment itself is a "killer" only if left untreated.

In fact, high blood pressure is actually one of the *easiest* of all ailments to detect, diagnose, and control, and learning whether or not you suffer from it could not be easier. All you need to do is check your blood pressure on a regular basis, and all that's required to accomplish this feat is a blood pressure cuff, your own or your doctor's. Three or four carefully monitored readings taken over the course of a day or two will give you a fair idea of where things stand.

As to hypertension's being a killer, this is undoubtedly true. Some experts label it the number one cause of death in the United States. High blood pressure can contribute to heart disease, hardening of the arteries, stroke, kidney damage, and several other nasty ailments, all of which are on the list of prominent killers. But *only* if you allow it to do so.

For the truth is that, of the countless ailments that rack the human machine, high blood pressure is one of the easiest to prevent, and one of the most responsive to treatment.

What's more, it is an ailment that for many people— a majority perhaps—can be kept partially or even fully under control simply by modifying one's lifestyle. The only step you must take to set the healing wheels in motion is to learn what these lifestyle modifications are, and to apply them to the fullest.

If you do this, if you learn about the many natural

options that are currently available to you for treating hypertension—and in this book we will tell you about them—chances are strong that your blood pressure will remain normal and under control for the rest of your natural life.


## How Prone Are You to High Blood Pressure?

Who gets hypertension?

A lot of people.

In the United States alone approximately forty-five to fifty million men and women suffer from the silent killer. That's *24 percent of the adult population*.

Among this group, roughly 75 percent have been officially diagnosed with the disease and 25 percent have not. That means that right this moment approximately eleven million people in the United States are cardiovascular casualties just waiting to happen.

Who gets the disease?

Since our circulatory apparatus tends to become less efficient as the years pass, older people are more likely to experience hypertension than young people. With each passing decade of the life cycle, a person's blood pressure creeps up a few points. More than 60 percent of people in their sixties have blood pressures above the normal range. Thus, while 120 over 80 may be a normal reading for a person under twenty years of age, 140 over 90 is more typical of someone in his or her seventies. With age comes elevated blood pressure. This is just part of the natural course of things, at least in the Western world.

What about heredity?

Individuals with a family history of hypertension are definitely more susceptible than those without. The degree of vulnerability depends on whether one or both parents suffer from the ailment.

If, for example, one of your parents has hypertension, your statistical chances of acquiring the disease are around fifty-fifty. If both parents have it, this ups the odds considerably.

Do not, however, let these figures make you fatalistic. Nothing is written in stone in these matters, and there are plenty of people with family histories full of hypertension who are free of the disease. Especially those who take proper care of themselves. Some researchers believe that we inherit a basic predisposition to high blood pressure, but that specific risk factors, such as obesity or lack of exercise, are needed to set it off.

What part does race play in this picture? African Americans of every age group have a proportionately higher chance of getting hypertension than whites. According to the National Institutes of Health, 50 percent of black people over the age of sixty-five in the United States suffer from hypertension, as opposed to 40 percent of white people in the same age category.

Genderwise, for people under the age of fifty high blood pressure is more apt to occur among men than women. After menopause, or more specifically after age fifty-five to sixty, women become more likely candidates than men. Among both sexes there is a gradual rise in blood pressure as the aging process unfolds.

## Natural Blood Pressure Control: What Makes It Such an Urgent Health Option?

For many years hypertension was looked upon as a purely physiological disease. Blood pressure levels, doctors observed, are established by a number of complex chemical processes that take place in our blood every moment of the day. And so doctors treated the disease in an appropriately physical way, using diuretics and synthesized chemical medicines to keep pressures normalized.

A number of these medicines were, and are, highly effective. They also tend to be costly, and in many cases they produce unpleasant side effects. Some blood pressure medications work well in controlling blood pressure but harm other parts of the body in the process. They may, for example, raise a person's blood-sugar levels, or increase blood fats.

Once a regimen of these drugs is started, moreover, patients are urged to continue on it for a lifetime. Weaning can be tricky business, and doctors warn of the perils. What's more, these medicines don't ever really cure the disease of hypertension. They simply control its harmful effects.

As the years passed, and as medical science began to discover that people's personal lifestyles affect their health in broad and hitherto unsuspected ways, both patients and physicians began to ask: Isn't it possible that high blood pressure is caused by more than a series of physiochemical reactions? Might not such lifestyle factors as diet, weight, emotions, personal habits, mental attitude, and environment also play a part? And if so, aren't there ways of addressing these factors, and of treating the disease in more holistic ways?

Time passed, and medical researchers began to understand the full extent to which lifestyle factors affect the development of hypertension. They began to see that through the control of these factors healing results could be gained.

What are these factors?

They are the very stuff of our day-to-day lives—the things that make us vital and human. They include:

- the ways we cope with the stress of daily living
- our social and emotional life
- our home and family life
- our personality type
- our exercise habits
- our weight
- our ability to relax
- our sleep patterns
- our vitamin and mineral intake
- our tendency to use (and misuse) addictive substances such as alcohol, caffeine, drugs, and cigarettes
- our diet: the foods and beverages we take into our bodies every day of our lives

All these lifestyle factors, medical researchers have come to understand, contribute in varying ways to the overall health of the cardiovascular system. Living right *does* make a difference, we now know. Natural and lifestyle factors *are* determinants in hypertension. The attitudes we develop toward taking charge of our living habits *do* affect our state of health—sometimes in a major way.

Hypertension, as one medical practitioner points out, is a disease caused to a large extent by the simple demands of modern living.

In this book we will introduce you to a number of easy-to-apply, nonmedical lifestyle improvements that you can start using right away, this very day, to gain control of your blood pressure. If your blood pressure is currently borderline high, and if you haven't yet gone on medication, you may find that by faithfully following the regimens laid out in this book, your problem will resolve itself on its own. If, on the other hand, you're already taking hypertensive medications, these techniques will serve as a powerful supplement to conventional medical treatment, and may even allow you to take smaller doses.

Or then again, if your blood pressure is already normal and you are anxious to keep it that way, the information offered in this book will help you to maintain the status quo. Prevention, as more and more Americans now understand, is the best of all medicines.

Whatever your particular situation happens to be, the lifestyle aids presented in this book will maximize the health of your circulatory system and increase your potential for leading a long, healthy life. Your part in the equation is to follow through on the methods presented here and to stick to them faithfully.

These methods work. Their value has been proven by millions of people the world over; they are tested, tried, and true. Adopt them as part of your routine of daily living and you will see the proof for yourself.

# 2

# What Is High Blood Pressure?

## What Is High Blood Pressure?

To answer this question it's first necessary to understand the workings of blood pressure in general.

Realize that the blood that pulses through our veins every moment of the day is propelled in rhythmic currents by a large and remarkably efficient mechanical pump—the heart. These currents make two major circuits.

The first circuit, referred to in medical language as *pulmonary circulation*, takes place when blood is pumped from the heart to the lungs, where it receives a rich supply of oxygen, and is then pumped back again to the heart.

The second circuit, termed *systemic circulation*, takes place when the aorta carries the oxygen-rich blood directly from the heart to the arteries. The arteries, in turn, transport the blood to smaller blood vessels, which pass it through to the capillaries, assuring that every cell of the body is bathed in this life-giving substance. Then the heart's pumping mechanism forces the blood back up through the veins to the heart. And so the process repeats itself day and night without cease. The sum total of this exquisite perpetual motion machine is known as the *cardiovascular system*.

Now, in order for this complex system to work at its maximum level, several factors are necessary.

One, the heart and lungs must function properly.

Two, the veins and arteries must be in good, flexible working condition, and their passageways must be clear.

Three, the pressure of the blood moving through the vessels must be in the right equilibrium to the vessel walls, neither too strong nor too weak. This pressure—*blood pressure*, we call it—is thus the force of the blood flowing along the vessels (and pounding against the walls of these vessels) as it moves through the body's network of arteries and veins.

Now let's suppose for a minute that one of these three variables is not working properly. Say for the sake of argument that the heart is pumping blood too quickly. This, in turn, causes the pressure in the blood vessels to rise.

Or perhaps some internal problem has caused the blood vessels to become constricted. In this instance, the narrowed vessels slow the flow, and pressure builds.

Think of a rubber hose. If you turn the nozzle on full blast, the pressure inside the hose increases. This is equivalent to what happens when the heart is beating rapidly. If you then squeeze the hose, this increases its internal pressure. Put the two together, increased flow and constricted passageways, and you have a working model of how high blood pressure operates in the human body.

Blood pressure, in short, is determined by the amount

of blood being pumped by the heart and the amount of resistance its flow encounters in the vessels.

Of course, people's blood pressures rises and falls throughout the day according to what they're doing. When we climb three flights of stairs to our apartment, when we cook a meal, when we take the dog for a brisk walk, our muscles require a greater supply of blood than when we're sitting in a chair. Our heart obliges by beating faster. This causes the blood to move more rapidly through the veins, and so blood pressure starts to rise.

Such elevation is not a case of high blood pressure per se. It is simply part of the normal rhythms that the cardiovascular system passes through during the day's alternating periods of exertion and rest. In a person with normal readings, blood pressure elevated by activity returns to an acceptable level as soon as these moments of effort are over, and it stays that way.

For some people, however, blood pressure levels slowly creep above the normal range and remain there for prolonged periods.

When this condition takes place, when blood pressure becomes chronically elevated and cannot be coaxed back to normal, we say that the person has high blood pressure. As soon as this condition is recognized, it's time to take action.

## What Causes High Blood Pressure?

If the truth be told, medical researchers are not entirely sure.

High blood pressure is a mysterious and complex ailment. Though years of research have gone into its study, and though we understand many of the mechanisms involved, doctors remain uncertain of what actually triggers hypertension at the deepest levels. Most likely it is the result of a complicated series of interactions between body systems, such as the adrenal glands, the autonomic nervous system, and the kidneys. Some research indicates that mechanisms in the brain may cause the problem. Other studies suggest that certain stress hormones are the culprit. Some medical researchers suspect that the heart itself plays a fundamental part. There are many theories.

To complicate matters, there are two types of high blood pressure.

The first, the variety that creeps up on people for no evident reason and that gradually becomes chronic, is known as *essential hypertension.* "Essential hypertension" is a technical way of defining high blood pressure that has no known cause. Or looked at in another way, it is blood pressure caused by a number of emotional, environmental, and physical variables, but with no single identifiable cause.

The second variety of high blood pressure, known as *secondary hypertension*, does not concern us directly in this book and is basically a complication caused by some specific other disease.

For example, Cushing's syndrome, sleep apnea, renovascular hypertension (narrowing of an artery in the kidneys), tumors in the adrenal glands, kidney disease, and other medical problems can all produce hypertensive symptoms. So, interestingly, can certain oral contraceptives, especially those that contain estrogen. If you are taking these medications, be sure and monitor your blood pressure closely, and keep your doctor apprised of any abnormal changes.

Finally, for many pregnant women blood pressure elevation can become a problem, though in most cases pressure tends to return to normal after the delivery. We will discuss the question of pregnancy and high blood pressure in a later section.

What percentage of people with high blood pressure suffer from secondary hypertension?

A very small one. If you have high blood pressure and if you are otherwise healthy, chances are around 95 percent that you have the essential variety.

This is bad news and good news. Bad because you have essential hypertension. Good because you don't have to struggle with another, more serious disease. And good because you have a medical problem you can do something about.

## What Effects Does High
## Blood Pressure Have on Your Health?

Here it is in a nutshell: If you suffer from untreated high blood pressure for a prolonged period of time, the effects of this dangerous disorder will gradually weaken several of your most important cardiovascular functions, making them prone to breakdown and disease.

## 1. The heart

First and foremost, there is the heart. When blood pressure is allowed to remain high over a period of years, the heart is obliged to work overtime and to pump blood more vigorously than it should.

As with any machine that is forced to work too long at too high a speed, the heart mechanism gradually begins to weaken. As time passes it may become enlarged, a condition known as *cardiomegaly*. Or the arteries may be constricted and blocked, causing blood flow to the heart to diminish, and small sections of heart muscle to waste away.

The person experiencing these negative changes may feel no symptoms whatsoever. Remember, hypertension is the silent killer. Then one day he or she typically begins to experience angina, a tightness or discomfort in the chest brought on by exertion or stress. Or an even more serious condition occurs: congestive heart failure, typified by shortness of breath, swelling, and fluid on the lung producing a hacking cough.

When these conditions strike they seem to be sudden and arbitrary. The truth is, they have been building up for years, decades even, due to the hidden ravages of hypertension.

## 2. The kidneys

The kidneys' major function is to filter the blood as it moves through its circuits, and to remove wastes that build up in the blood. They then dump these toxic residues into the urine for excretion.

If this blood flow to the kidneys is reduced through

hardening of its vessels caused by hypertension, the toxins will no longer be eliminated properly and will remain in the blood, eventually causing a state of poisoning known as *uremia*. The consequences of this condition can include diminished kidney efficiency, oxygen-starved tissue, and—worst-case scenario—kidney failure.

Today, with effective forms of self-care and medication, hypertension-related kidney problems are easy to treat, and most people's renal function can be restored to normal—but only if their condition is not allowed to progress too far.

### 3. The brain

Over the long term, untreated high blood pressure weakens the walls of the cerebral blood vessels and may induce a thickening in the lining of the vessel walls, causing hardening of the arteries, or *atherosclerosis*. These changes create the conditions for a *stroke*.

Technically speaking, a stroke is damage done to the brain by the leaking or rupture of blood vessels, which in turn causes an interruption of blood supply to the brain. When blood is not brought to the cerebral tissues, their supply of oxygen is cut off, and the deprived areas begin to die.

There are three basic kinds of stroke:

*Cerebral thrombosis* accounts for almost 50 percent of strokes. It is caused by clots that build up over time in the artery walls of the brain and block the flow of blood to tissue.

*Cerebral embolisms* are triggered by clots as well,

but usually by clots transported to the brain from other parts of the body, such as the heart.

Finally, a *cerebral hemorrhage* occurs when a vessel suddenly ruptures or slowly leaks. The result is local or generalized bleeding in the brain.

While the results of a stroke can be devastating, the degree of damage that follows depends on the variety of stroke that has occurred, and on the part of the brain affected. In some instances a stroke can be so small it goes unnoticed. Some people experience a number of small strokes over an extended period of time and have few if any symptoms to show for it. For others the results of a single stroke can be catastrophic, producing mental deficits, physical handicaps, paralysis, coma, and, not infrequently, death.

Approximately one out of three strokes is fatal. And significantly, hypertension is considered by medical authorities to be the number one cause of stroke.

## 4. The eyes

Visitors to the doctor's office are often surprised to learn that under certain conditions a physician can discover evidence of high blood pressure by examining the eyes.

Why? Because if blood pressure is elevated for a long period of time, the small veins in the eye are affected, and begin to wither and erode. These afflicted veins can be observed by any trained medical practitioner.

The area of the eye most commonly affected by hypertension is the retina. The harm to this tender area may be mild—most of the time this is the case. But occasionally there can be severe damage, causing a detached retina or retinal hemorrhages.

Both conditions can ultimately lead to blindness.

## 5. The arteries

"Hardening of the arteries" is a high-recognition term in our society, and so is its technical name, *atherosclerosis*. But not everyone is certain what it means.

In brief, hardening of the arteries is a progressive thickening in the blood vessels that occurs naturally in all of us as we age, but that is accelerated in those with elevated blood pressure. As the blood of a hypertensive person flows through the vessels year after year at higher pressures than normal, the walls of the vessels slowly become leathery and lose their flexibility. The vessels also tend to shrink, narrow, and constrict.

If this narrowing goes undiagnosed and untreated, unpleasant things start to happen. If, for example, the narrowing is centered in the legs, the legs become deprived of their normal quota of blood. Leg pains, cramps, and difficulty in walking are the results. If the vessels in and around the heart are constricted, cardiovascular ailments, such as angina, can follow. If constriction takes place in the vessels inside the brain, stroke becomes a possibility.

Happily, hardening of the arteries, if caught in time, is reversible, both through the use of medication and with proper diet, exercise, and lifestyle.

## Personal Risk Factors That
## Lead to High Blood Pressure

The items on the list of risk factors below are health-threatening only if you let them be.

Weight, for example. Maintaining an ideal weight is, of course, not a risk factor for hypertension, but rather a means of avoiding the disease. Allowing one-self to become obese, on the other hand, is a risk factor par excellence.

The entries on the list below, therefore, though typically referred to as risk factors, are "risky" only if allowed to take a negative course. Except for genetics and gender, each of these factors can be controlled and modified in a positive way, and each factor can, if properly channeled, become an ally rather than a liability.

Read the listings with a careful eye. Consider the implications of each, especially in the context of your own health. Then ask yourself: How can I use each of these factors to improve my health in general, and to lower my potential for hypertension in particular?

We will discuss each of these risk factors more thoroughly in the chapters that follow.

### 1. Genetics

As mentioned, if one or both of your parents suffer from hypertension, your odds of acquiring the condition at some point in life are increased. Having a brother or a sister with problematic blood pressure increases the likelihood even more.

Thus, if you have a family history of hypertension, and if you have not been checked out in this department for a while, it's a good idea to visit your doctor right away and get a set of up-to-date blood pressure readings.

Remember again, though: As far as genetics is concerned nothing is ever definitive.

Though biologically you may be linked to your family tree, you are also your own person with a distinctive constitution and unique set of genes. The course your health takes over the years will be entirely your own, and there are many personal actions you can take right now to countermand whatever inborn tendencies threaten your cardiovascular system.

Genetics, in this sense, is a tendency rather than an absolute, a kind of warning sign along the path of life that reads: "Potential danger. Take all appropriate steps to avoid." Follow this advice with proper living habits, and chances are that whatever predisposition you have toward hypertension will be offset.

## 2. Gender

When young, men appear to suffer from hypertension more frequently than women. After the age of fifty-five to sixty, women acquire the disorder more commonly than men.

Interestingly, there is evidence to suggest that elderly women tolerate hypertension better than men. In general, women suffer cardiac problems less frequently than males, and biologically they seem better equipped than men to endure higher blood pressures for longer lengths of time.

### 3. Weight

Obese people tend to have higher blood pressures than those whose weight is appropriate to their size and bone structure. According to the famous Framingham Heart Study, men and women who are 20 percent above their ideal weight have an *eight times greater* chance of suffering elevated blood pressure than those who are at their ideal weight.

Individuals with borderline and mild hypertension often discover that simply by dropping extra pounds they can reduce their blood pressure substantially, sometimes to the range of normalcy.

As far as high blood pressure is concerned, weight matters.

### 4. Alcohol use

For some years it was argued that people who misuse alcohol have a great deal of stress in their lives. Therefore, it was believed, stress is the cause of the high blood pressure, not alcohol.

Today medical researchers are reasonably sure that a direct physical relationship exists between alcohol consumption and elevated pressure readings. Indeed, in a small population of hypertensive persons, alcohol appears to be the *primary* cause of the disease. Studies show that when members of this high-risk group cut back on alcohol consumption, or when they stop drinking entirely, their blood pressure returns to normal.

Nothing is absolute here. There are plenty of heavy drinkers with normal blood pressure, and plenty of nondrinkers with high blood pressure. On the other hand, overindulgence in alcohol is harmful to the body in a number of ways, each of which wears down physical resistance and makes people more vulnerable than usual to ailments they might otherwise not acquire—hypertension included.

## 5. Stress

Although it is a difficult factor to measure with scientific precision, stress—along with anxiety, nervousness, frustration, and all the kindred emotions—clearly plays a role in the development of hypertension. Studies have determined time and again that Type A personalities, those persons who are aggressive, impatient, quickly frustrated, and easily angered, are approximately *twice as likely* to suffer from coronary problems as the less driven and less competitive Type Bs.

For some people, then, stress is a key factor in cardiovascular health, and simply by applying relaxation and meditation techniques they are able to bring their pressure down to manageable levels.

We will discuss the matter of stress and hypertension at length in subsequent chapters.

## 6. Smoking

For many years it has been known that when you smoke a cigarette your blood pressure goes up. But this increase is temporary. Several minutes later your pressure returns to normal.

Thus it is difficult to pin anything directly on smoking as a cause of hypertension.

At the same time, we know that smoking is one of the most dangerous acts a person can indulge in, and that it imposes an amazingly wide assortment of ill effects on the cardiovascular system. Those who suffer from untreated hypertension already have an increased potential for developing heart and lung disease. By smoking they radically heighten this potential, raising it from a possibility to a probability—and beyond.

## 7. Lack of exercise

If you already have high blood pressure, or if a family history worries you for the future, there is considerable clinical evidence that a robust program of aerobic exercise and systematic cardiovascular conditioning can postpone the effects of, and in some cases circumvent, a predisposition toward this disease.

Lack of exercise, on the other hand, with all the sedentary habits that go with it, appears to encourage high blood pressure, along with a general state of ill health.

The heart, the lungs, the circulation, the digestive system all prosper from vigorous workouts, and all wither without it. Inveterate couch potatoes should be warned: By remaining physically inactive you are dramatically increasing your potential not just for hypertension but for heart disease, stroke, and a host of other heart and lung ailments.

As far as our bodies go, disuse is abuse.

## 8. Age

Your blood pressure will probably never be lower than during the first few weeks after you are born. After that it's all downhill.

Well, not exactly.

As time passes, and as we live through our youth, middle age, early old age, and late old age, blood pressure readings tend to rise. This is a natural biological process common to all human beings, but one that should be carefully watched.

After forty years of age every man and woman should have a regular blood pressure checkup several times a year. Stick to this regimen faithfully and you can't go wrong.

## 9. Blood cholesterol levels

Cholesterol is a yellowish, waxy, fatty substance that is found in many organs of the body, and that plays a critical role in the health of our cells.

For reasons not entirely understood, in many people the production of this essential ingredient gets out of hand, and it ends up as deposits on the walls of the blood vessels, eventually blocking the flow of blood and contributing to hardening of the arteries.

Although the actual relationship between high cholesterol and hypertension is subject to argument, we know from many studies that people with high blood pressure tend to have high cholesterol counts as well.

Bottom line, then: If you have high blood pressure *and* high cholesterol your chance of developing coronary disease is a good deal greater than if you have normal blood pressure and cholesterol count.

Fortunately, high cholesterol can be controlled. Many people take care of the problem through diet alone.

## 10. Diet

Many medical experts believe that the single most powerful natural aid we have in our war chest against hypertension is diet control.

Natural diet control in this context means two things:

- what we eat
- what we don't eat

Of course, there is a great deal of balderdash today concerning wonder diets and miracle supplements, and to a certain extent you may feel jaded from the many false claims.

But don't lose heart. Because the fact is that by eating certain kinds of foods, avoiding other kinds of foods, and adopting a diet especially formatted to control hypertension, you may be able to keep your blood pressure down without recourse to drugs.

When all is said and done, a proper diet is potentially your greatest ally in the battle against hypertension. The final parts of this book will go into the question of hypertension and nutrition in depth.

## How Do You Know if You Have High Blood Pressure?

Is there really *no* perceptible symptom of high blood pressure?

In most cases, yes. But there are exceptions.

Basically, there are five levels of hypertension:

- borderline
- mild
- moderate
- severe
- very severe

Individuals at the first three levels, borderline, mild, and moderate, tend to remain asymptomatic. There are exceptions, but not many.

Severe and very severe hypertension, which, roughly speaking, include readings of 180 over 110 and above—how these numbers work will be explained as we go—can indeed produce overt symptoms. When pressures reach these extreme limits, unpleasant reactions appear, sometimes with a vengeance. Symptoms of severe hypertension include:

- recurring headache
- blurred vision or sudden lack of vision
- extreme dizziness and vertigo
- ringing in the ears
- undue fatigue, usually accompanied by irritability and malaise
- shortness of breath
- chest pains
- persistent nosebleeds

Of these symptoms, headaches are probably the most common, and they are often of an incredibly painful and throbbing kind.

Blurred eyesight, or even loss of vision, can occur

when blood vessels burst in the back of the eye due to pressure buildup in the veins over long periods of time.

Dizziness and ringing in the ears are frequent symptoms when pressures soar. In severe cases of dizziness a person may be unable to stand up without falling.

Shortness of breath, a feeling of heaviness in the chest, and swelling in various parts of the body, especially the legs, can all signal congestive heart failure. If you see any evidence of these, go to a physician immediately.

Nosebleeds are a particular cause for concern when they occur frequently, when they are difficult to stop, and when they happen in concert with one or more of the symptoms listed above.

Severe hypertension is often considered an emergency condition and should never be neglected. Even if the problem turns out to be something other than hypertension, experiencing two or more of the symptoms listed above should be cause for concern under any circumstances, especially for men and women over forty.

What about persons with borderline, mild, and moderate high blood pressures? How are they to know they have blood pressure woes?

As we've seen, most people in these categories can go for years and never know anything is amiss. For these people—and this means the vast majority of us—there is only one way to get to the heart of the matter. Have your blood pressure taken.

## Measuring Your Blood Pressure

When you visit your physician for a physical exam, one of the first procedures he or she performs is to take your blood pressure. If you are over forty years old, the doctor will probably take several readings, one on each arm and perhaps a reading lying down and standing up as well.

Why both arms? Isn't blood pressure fairly even on both sides of the body?

In general, yes, though readings on the right arm tend to be a bit higher than on the left. What the doctor is looking for here is imbalance: that is, any significant discrepancy between readings on the body's right side and left. Too large a gap between sides can mean that the aorta, the central blood vessel that leads from the heart, is unnaturally constricted.

To measure your blood pressure the doctor uses a stethoscope and a special measuring device known as a *sphygmomanometer*. This ingenious machine consists of a mercury-filled tube (much like an ordinary thermometer) calibrated from base to top with millimeter (mm) readings and attached to an inflatable cloth cuff via a rubber hose.

First, the cloth cuff is wrapped around the upper arm. The doctor pumps air into the cuff by squeezing an attached rubber bulb. The cuff is inflated until the column of mercury reaches 190 to 200 mm Hg in the tube. (Hg is the symbol for mercury.) At this point all blood movement in the arm is cut off by the tightness of the cuff.

The cuff is now slowly deflated and the blood in the arm starts to flow again.

As the air gradually escapes the cuff, the doctor listens for a pulse through the stethoscope placed on the inside crook of the patient's arm. At the moment when the pulse begins, the doctor checks the numerical reading on the mercury tube. In a person with normal blood pressure this reading will be around 120 or 130 mm Hg. In someone with high blood pressure it could be as high as 160 or 170 mm Hg. The number where the pulse is first heard through the stethoscope marks the so-called *systolic*, or upper, blood pressure reading.

The doctor continues to listen through the stethoscope. The sound of the pulse increases in intensity for several moments, then it slowly dies away. The point at which the sound of the pulse stops entirely marks the *diastolic*, or lower, blood pressure reading.

Thus, in a person with a blood pressure reading of 120 over 80, the 120 represents the systolic or upper pressure, the 80 the diastolic or lower. This reading is verbally expressed as "one-twenty over eighty." It is written as: 120/80.

A good mnemonic device for remembering the easily forgettable sequence of systolic on top, diastolic on the bottom is to think of the phrase *simple dimple*. First comes the *s* in *simple*, standing for systolic, then the *d* in *dimple*, for diastolic.

What do the systolic and diastolic pressures represent?

Physiologically, the systolic pressure occurs at the moment when blood is propelled from the heart to the arteries. Understand that blood does not flow through our veins like a calm stream meandering its way across a meadow. The mechanism is more akin to waves breaking on the shore. These waves pulse ahead in rhythmic surges, each surge produced by a beat of the heart. Measured in terms of pressure, each of these heartbeats represents the systolic, or upper, reading.

Then the wave recedes, as it were, and a brief resting period follows. This moment of inactivity and pause between heartbeats represents the diastolic, or lower, pressure reading.

The systolic reading, therefore, gauges blood pressure at the moment the heart is beating. The diastolic measures pressure while the heart rests.

What would a perfect blood pressure be?

Conventional wisdom has it that 120/80 is ideal. But this is a ballpark figure and in many ways an arbitrary one. In European countries norms are higher, and a reading of 140/85 would raise few medical eyebrows.

What's more, a person's blood pressure is continually changing, depending on what activities the person is involved in during the day. Moments of physical or mental stress cause pressures to go way up, moments of rest drop it down. Even people with excellent blood pressures rarely maintain the 120/80 ideal for more than a few moments every day.

Conventional wisdom also has it that ideal blood pressure depends on a person's age. As we've seen, the older people get, the higher their pressures tend to go. A reading of 150/92 in a man of eighty might be considered well within the realm of the acceptable by many physicians. In a man of twenty-one it would be instant cause for concern.

Yet even here there are no certainties. For years higher blood pressures were considered normal in older persons. Today's thinking holds that high blood pressure is harmful for people at any age, and that there is no biological mandate telling us we *must* become hypertensive just because we are up in years.

Yet even while it's difficult to pinpoint an ideal blood pressure, modern medicine has established measurement perimeters that are accepted by most health care professionals in the United States, and that provide reasonable criteria for judging the health of one's blood pressure.

These perimeters are as follows:

- A reading of 120mm Hg over 80mm Hg is considered *ideal*.
- A reading of 130 to 139mm Hg over 80 to 84 mm Hg is considered *high normal* blood pressure.
- A reading of 140 to 159 mm Hg over 90 to 99 mm Hg is *mild hypertension* (known as Stage 1 hypertension).
- A reading of 160 to 179 mm Hg over 100 to 109 mm Hg is *moderate hypertension* (known as Stage 2 hypertension).
- A reading of 180 to 209 mm Hg over 110 to 119 mm Hg is *high hypertension* (known as Stage 3 hypertension).
- A reading of 210 mm Hg or above over 120 mm Hg or above is *severe hypertension* (known as Stage 4 hypertension).

NOTE: These figures are based on two or more blood pressure readings. They are taken from information published by the National Heart, Lung and Blood Institute, National Institutes of Health.

Which is the more important of the two readings, the systolic (upper) or the diastolic (lower)?

This is also a controversial question and one on which not all doctors agree.

All things considered, most clinicians will probably tell you that an elevated resting, or diastolic, pulse is more worrisome than an elevated systolic. When visiting your doctor, if your blood pressure clocks in at, say, 140/100, this is more likely to trigger concern than a reading of 160/88.

Why? Because the systolic or upper reading has a wider and more flexible range than the diastolic. The moment we become stressed or highly active, the moment we begin vacuuming the house or run to catch a bus, it's perfectly natural for the systolic reading to shoot up. In times of great physical effort it's not unusual for the systolic to elevate 50 points or more. Serious weight lifters making a big lift sometimes record a systolic of over 300 mm Hg!

The diastolic is less volatile than the systolic, and tends to go up or down a few points at most, even in times of stress and activity.

Yet with the diastolic a little is a lot. According to the Framingham Heart Study, lowering the diastolic pressure by as little as 2 mm Hg over an extended period of time can result in a 6 percent reduction in risk of stroke.

That's the good news.

The bad news is that if your diastolic *increases* just 2 or 3 mm for an extended period of time, the reverse situation occurs, and risk of stroke goes up commensurately.

Still and all, don't assume that one part of your reading is ultimately more significant than the other. The Framingham study suggests that both pressures, systolic and diastolic, are generally of equal importance, and that as we age the impact of the diastolic pressure on heart disease risk actually declines while the importance of the systolic increases.

All things considered, then, one should not favor either side of a blood pressure reading. Better to consider the reading as a whole and go from there.

## Other Clinical Methods for Diagnosing High Blood Pressure

Are there other measurable indications of high blood pressure besides the overt symptoms that appear in severe cases and the readings on the blood pressure cuff?

Yes, but they are less direct and must be ferreted out through inquiry and examination. When your physician examines you, he or she will always be looking for these subtle indicators that can suggest, though not necessarily confirm, blood pressure complications.

To begin, a doctor will conduct an oral medical interview, asking you questions about your medical history. The doctor will want to know the health of your parents and siblings, your personal health habits, and your current state of fitness and well-being. Have you lost or gained weight lately? What medications (including birth control pills) are you currently taking? Any unusual symptoms? Do you smoke or drink? If so, how much?

A physical exam follows, with procedures that implicitly probe for hypertension.

Doctors may, for example, palpate your abdomen, looking for dark-colored stretch marks that indicate possible adrenal hyperactivity. Protrusions in the abdomen can indicate an enlarged kidney or an aneurysm of the aorta, both hypertension-related conditions.

Stand-out blood vessels on the arms and legs will be looked at for signs of arteriosclerosis. The eyes will be studied for burst or twisted blood vessels. The examiner will listen carefully to the heart for murmurs, irregular beats, and enlargement, all possible indicators of chronic hypertension. After you reach age forty, most doctors will also require you to take a standard electrocardiogram (EKG) to monitor the health of the heart in general, and to search for signs of injury from past, possibly undetected heart problems.

Besides a direct physical examination physicians will also want to run several tests that have a bearing on possible hypertension. These include:

• *Blood creatine or urea.* This test determines if kidney problems are present.

• *Blood cholesterol.* High cholesterol can be an indicator of clogged veins and possible hypertension.

• *Chest X ray.* From a cardiovascular perspective, X rays help determine if there is any enlargement of the heart (a possible sign of hypertension).

• *Urinanalysis.* This test searches for indications of diabetes (a condition that often accompanies high blood pressure).

• *Blood potassium.* This test looks for tumors in the adrenal glands.

These and several other laboratory tests may be ordered, depending on the patient's age and state of health. When all is said and done, however, the bottom-line indicator for essential hypertension is and always has been the reading you see on the blood pressure cuff. Nine times out of ten this reading is all you'll need.

## Taking Your Own Blood Pressure

For people with normal and elevated blood pressures alike, an investment of as little as thirty-five dollars can buy a home-use blood pressure cuff that provides reasonably accurate readings at any time, day or night.

No doubt you've seen these devices for sale. They're everywhere these days, in department stores, mall shops, pharmacies, health care catalogs. The cheaper models require you to pump up the pressure in the cuff yourself with the ubiquitous rubber bulb. More expensive models do the pumping for you. With the self-inflating variety, all that's needed on your part is to wrap the cuff around your arm and push a button. The machine does the rest, inflating the cuff to the proper pressure, deflating it slowly, and giving you the systolic/diastolic reading automatically on a digital readout.

Many people prefer the self-inflating model, not only because it's easier to use, but because squeezing the bulb to inflate the cuff can make your blood pressure rise a small but real percentage as well, skewing the accuracy of the readings. In today's market you can find self-inflating models for under fifty dollars. Check magazines like *Consumer Reports* for the most reliable models.

How accurate are home-use blood pressure cuffs?

Fairly accurate, though certainly not as precise as the more costly and better-made sphygmomanometer that your physician uses.

A good way of determining how precise the readings on your home-use meter are is to take it with you to your doctor's office next time you go—or, for that matter, to any location where blood pressure readings are done (free blood pressure stations are frequently set up as a community service at malls, street fairs, and local hospitals).

After your pressure is measured with the sphygmomanometer, check it against the readings on your own machine. You won't get an identical reading this way, as your blood pressure varies from moment to moment. But if your home-use machine's numbers are close to the ones on the professional model by a factor of, say, plus or minus 5 mm Hg, you know you're using a machine you can trust.

## A Few Helps and Hints for Taking Your Own Blood Pressure

1. Before you start taking your blood pressure, sit for several minutes and relax. One of the advantages of taking blood pressure at home is that you are less nervous than in the physician's office. In fact, a number of people experience a phenomenon known as "white coat hypertension," whereby they register abnormally high

blood pressures *only* in a doctor's office. The rest of the time their pressures are normal. Using a home machine is the perfect antidote.

2. When pumping up your blood pressure cuff, don't make sudden movements. In fact, don't move at all, and don't talk at all. The slightest exertion can skew your readings.

3. If you are using a manually inflatable cuff, have another person do the pumping. Allowing someone else to do the work for you cuts down your activity and gives you a more reliable reading.

4. Take readings on both your right arm and your left. Expect the right arm reading to be slightly higher than the left. Any extreme gaps in the readings between right and left should be reported to your physician.

5. If you take more than one reading on the same arm, wait at least thirty seconds between measurements. If you take a reading too soon, blood will remain constricted in the veins, and you won't get an accurate figure.

6. Physicians often take more than one blood pressure reading when a patient comes into the office. They may take one reading at the beginning of the appointment and one at the end. In this way a mean blood pressure average is ascertained. You can accomplish the same goal using your own cuff. Take several readings over, say, a twenty-minute period, then average them. This will give you a pretty fair picture of what your blood pressure is doing on this particular day.

7. If you wish to establish a long-term picture of how your blood pressure behaves, keep a daily readings

chart for several months. On a pad or sheet of paper, mark down the figure of each reading and date it. In this way you, and if necessary your doctor, will have a clear picture of how your blood pressure is behaving over an extended period of time.

8. Be careful of what some people call home blood pressure fixation. The downside of owning one's own meter is that in some cases people become so concerned with their blood pressure that they take readings every hour or so, worrying themselves miserable each time the numbers go a little too high. Not everyone experiences this fixation, of course, but some do. The best way to avoid it is simply to set yourself limits. One set of readings in the morning and one set at night is enough to give anyone an accurate picture. More than this becomes counterproductive.

## High Blood Pressure and Pregnancy: What You Should Know

Women who experience moderate blood pressure elevations during pregnancy need not worry about this condition as long as their doctor is apprised of the situation, and the pressure is monitored carefully. In some cases the pregnancy itself raises the mother's blood pressure. In other instances the pregnancy unmasks a previously hidden condition.

Treatment usually consists of natural methods, such as salt-free meals, special diets, exercise, and weight reduction. Under certain conditions antihypertensive medicines will be given, though most physicians prefer not to take this route unless it's absolutely necessary. A majority of women who suffer from mild to moderate hypertension get through their pregnancies without undue problems.

A small number of expectant mothers, however, develop serious high blood pressure in the last trimester—a condition that causes palpable symptoms such as edema (swelling) in the ankles and legs, headaches, spots in front of the eyes, sudden weight gain, and more. The systolic pressure can climb 30 mm Hg points or higher with this condition, the diastolic 15 mm Hg or more.

These symptoms are due to a condition known as toxemia or preeclampsia. No one is certain why some women develop this affliction, though it is known that women in their first pregnancy, women bearing twins, and women with diabetes have an elevated chance of acquiring it. Developing this condition in one's first pregnancy is by no means a guarantee that it will be repeated in the second. In fact, toxemia tends not to return in subsequent pregnancies.

How serious is toxemia/preeclampsia?

It depends on how high the blood pressure goes. In mild cases bed rest under the supervision of a physician is the treatment of choice. More severe cases require medication and perhaps hospitalization.

Possible effects of untreated preeclampsia include premature birth, low birth weight, kidney failure in the mother, and, in extreme cases, convulsions in the mother and death for the child.

But take heart. As long as you put yourself under a

doctor's care, toxemia/preeclampsia can be controlled. In most cases the condition is temporary. A few days after your baby enters the world, the hypertension will most likely fade away, never to reappear. Do be careful, though: hypertension during any part of the pregnancy cycle is nothing to ignore. At the first sign of blood pressure elevation, see your doctor.

## Medication: What Are Today's Best Options?

While this is a book about the natural treatment of hypertension, and while any lengthy discussion of the mechanism of blood pressure medicines is beyond our scope, it's also important for your own self-care to gain a working familiarity with the antihypertension drugs that are currently on the market, and to acquire a basic awareness concerning the pros and cons of each. In this way, if it should become necessary for you to begin a regimen of blood pressure medication, you will approach your treatment from a position of knowledge rather than ignorance, and that's the most important thing any of us can do for our own state of health.

The following section offers a kind of crash course in blood pressure medication, with thumbnail sketches of the most popular antihypertensive drug families in use today *just in case* you need them someday.

## How Safe Are Blood Pressure Medications?

If your grandfather or aunt or an aging friend suffered from a bout of hypertension in the past, and if that person was treated with antihypertensive medications, it's very possible that he or she has already regaled you with horror stories of vertigo, pounding headaches, diarrhea, depression, impotence, and so forth, all caused by a high blood pressure prescription.

While all this was true at one time, substantial strides have been made over the past decades in improving blood pressure medications, and today many of the best preparations produce far fewer side effects than before.

This is not to say that antihypertensives are side-effect free. They're not. In some cases side effects linger and cause discomfort. All things considered, though, the situation has improved, and if you're going to be treated medically for high blood pressure, this is the best time in medical history for it to happen.

What are the major families of blood pressure lowering medications?

There are six of them, as follows:

### 1. Diuretics

*Profile.* Diuretics are prescribed to rid the body of excessive water retention, often in cases of congestive heart disease. When given for hypertension, diuretics are frequently prescribed in concert with other drugs. Continual use of these preparations for at least two to three weeks is necessary to see results. But be warned: Taking diuretics over an extended period of time can in some cases cause severe potassium and magnesium loss, along with impaired water balance. Mineral loss is covered in the section on diuretic side effects below.

*Mechanism of action.* While most blood pressure medications work by preventing the constriction of blood vessels or promoting their dilation, diuretics function in a different way, removing salts (mostly sodium and potassium) from the urine, speeding up the elimination of salt and water through urination, and thus reducing the fluid and salt retention throughout the body that increases blood pressure. Diuretics, in short, perform much the same function in your system as a low-salt diet.

*Side effects.* Generally speaking, diuretics tend to produce a larger number of side effects than other blood pressure medications. These include:

• *Frequent urination.* As with diuretic foods like watermelon or coffee, prescription diuretics increase the volume and frequency of urination. As time passes, this response tends to decrease.

• *Rashes.* Skin problems sometimes occur with diuretics, as they can with many blood pressure medications. This side effect tends to occur in a relatively small number of patients.

• *Increased blood sugar.* Certain diuretics elevate blood sugar levels. For this reason they are not advisable for use by diabetics or by people who have been diagnosed with prediabetic conditions. If you have trouble in this area be sure and tell your doctor before he or she prescribes any antihypertensive medication.

• *Increased cholesterol.* There is evidence that over time diuretics can slightly increase both the cholesterol and triglyceride levels in the blood, thereby reducing the effectiveness of the body's natural clotting agents and making a person more vulnerable to cardiovascular episodes. Be watchful here if heart disease is a problem. Again, check with your doctor.

• *Reduction of certain minerals in the system.* Both magnesium and potassium are depleted by diuretic preparations. Reactions to this depletion may include missed heartbeats and arrhythmia (irregular heartbeat). Mineral supplements and diets rich in magnesium and potassium are useful for correcting this deficiency. Potassium-rich foods include bananas, green leafy vegetables, oranges, grapefruit, whole grains, sunflower seeds, potatoes, lean meats, and dried apricots. Magnesium-rich foods include green leafy vegetables (magnesium is an essential element of chlorophyll), wheat germ, apples, almonds, figs, corn, and soybeans.

• *Gout.* Certain diuretics can increase the levels of uric acid in the blood, producing the very painful disease of gout. If any symptoms of gout begin to appear while you are on diuretics, speak with your physician immediately. The primary symptom of gout is the sudden development of a red, swollen, extremely tender joint, usually the joint in the big toe.

## 2. Beta-blockers

*Profile.* Originally developed by Nobel Prize–winner James Black as a heart medication, beta-blockers can in many instances keep blood pressure and heart problems under control, especially chest pains and effort-induced angina. From a circulatory standpoint, beta-blockers are used to counteract mild to moderate hypertension. In some cases they help fight migraine headaches as well. Continual use for ten days to two weeks is necessary to see results. Maximum effectiveness is usually reached after six to eight weeks.

*Mechanism of action.* Beta-receptors are sensory nerve cells located throughout the cardiovascular system and specifically in the areas of the heart, lungs, and vein walls. Their job is to receive the nerve and chemical messages that speed up heartbeat and tell the blood vessels to constrict. Beta-blockers work by impeding the reception of these messages, preventing the heart from beating too quickly and the veins from constricting—and thereby lowering blood pressure.

*Side effects.* Possible side effects of beta-blockers include:

• *Fatigue.* Since the beta-blockers slow down the heart and pulse, they also tend to produce a slowing of the system as a whole. This effect is experienced as undue tiredness and lethargy. For this reason, beta-blockers are not always the medicine of choice for athletes and manual laborers.

• *Orthostatic hypotension.* A condition of sudden drop in blood pressure, resulting from standing up suddenly. (See the reference to orthostatic hypotension in the section on alpha-blocker side effects below.)

• *Cold extremities.* Beta-blockers constrict the peripheral blood vessels, causing a sense of coldness and clamminess in the hands and feet.

• *Reduction in achieving cardiovascular fitness.* By lowering the heart rate and keeping it there, beta-blockers make it extremely difficult, if not impossible, for people who participate in serious aerobic exercise to bring their heart rates up enough to receive maximum benefits. Athletes especially find that a lowered heartbeat keeps them from performing at their maximum.

• *Depression.* One study revealed that close to a quarter of patients taking beta-blockers were on antidepressant medications.

• *Impaired sexual function.* Decreased sexual drive is not uncommon for men using beta-blockers. Impotence and difficulty in achieving erection are relatively common.

## 3. Alpha-blockers

*Profile.* Alpha-blockers are often the first drug of choice in mild to moderate cases of hypertension. They may also be prescribed along with other antihypertension drugs to treat severe cases. Continual use for four to six weeks is necessary to achieve maximum effectiveness. If you suffer from depression and/or if you are taking antidepressive drugs, tell your doctor before using an alpha-blocker.

*Mechanism of action.* The walls of human blood vessels are lined with many *alpha-receptors*, highly sensitive nerve cells designed to receive the chemical and nerve commands that tell the blood vessels when to tighten and constrict. Alpha-blockers inhibit these receptors, causing the vessels to relax and to remain in an expanded state. This expansion allows the blood to flow more freely, and the pressure to drop. There is some evidence that alpha-blockers also reduce blood cholesterol levels.

*Side effects.* Possible side effects of alpha-blockers include:

• *Orthostatic or postural hypotension.* This is a type of low (not high) blood pressure related to body posture. When standing up, people prone to orthostatic hypotension experience sudden dizziness, faintness, and loss of balance. Those just starting on alpha-blockers often experience orthostatic hypotension the first half hour after taking the drug—the so-called first dose effect. Although harmless in itself, orthostatic hypotension can cause patients to take sudden and severe falls. A well-managed dosage schedule, beginning with small doses and gradually increasing the amounts, usually keeps this problem under control.

• *Drowsiness.* Be careful driving or performing dangerous work while taking these drugs.

• *Dry mouth.* A common side effect of many medications.

• *Constipation, nasal congestion, sleep disturbances.*

## 4. ACE inhibitors

*Profile.* Though on the market for little more than a decade, ACE inhibitors rank among the most popular of all blood pressure drugs. They are generally used to treat mild to moderate hypertension. When they are used to treat severe hypertension, a diuretic or second hypertensive medication is usually prescribed. Continual use for two to three weeks is necessary to reach maximum effectiveness. On the whole, ACE inhibitors cause a low incidence of adverse side effects.

*Mechanism of action.* Angiotensin Converting Enzyme Inhibitors (ACE Inhibitors) work in the following way: *Angiotensin converting enzyme* converts a substance called angiotensin I into a substance called angiotensin II. The principal job angiotensin II performs in the body is to constrict blood vessels. When this conversion process is blocked and when angiotensin II production is inhibited, the blood vessels remain open and dilated. Blood pressure then drops. ACE inhibitors are also used for treating heart failure.

*Side effects.* Possible side effects include:

• *Dizziness, headache, and fatigue.* All three of these reactions occur in less than 5 percent of patients.

• *Orthostatic hypotension.* A sudden drop in blood pressure, resulting from standing up suddenly. (See the reference to orthostatic hypotension in the section on alpha-blocker side effects, above.)

• *Skin rash.* Again, only a small percent of patients experience this effect.

• *Dry cough.* Perhaps the most common side effect of ACE inhibitors, the cough is more an irritation than a major problem.

### 5. Calcium channel blockers

*Profile.* Calcium channel blockers are a dual-use medication, effective both for controlling hypertension and for counteracting several types of angina. While there has been some controversy concerning the long-term safety of these drugs, physicians still prescribe them today on a regular basis, though perhaps not as frequently as other antihypertensives. If you have diabetes or impaired liver or kidney function, be sure and report this fact to your physician before starting a regimen of calcium channel blockers. Patients as a rule take calcium channel blockers for two to four weeks before they experience optimum results.

*Mechanism of action.* In order for muscle cells in the arteries to contract, a certain amount of calcium must be present to catalyze the process. This calcium reaches the muscles and veins through discrete "channels," or passageways, in the cell membranes. Calcium channel blockers plug these passageways, interfering with the transportation of calcium to the veins, and thus inhibiting vessel constriction.

*Side effects.* The side effects of calcium channel blockers tend to be relatively benign. They include:

• *Constipation.* A sizable percentage of people on calcium channel blockers suffer from constipation. Since calcium blockers slow the contraction of intestinal muscles, they interfere with peristalsis, and thus with elimination. For people who suffer from this side effect, a diet rich in vegetables, fruits, and fermented foods like sauerkraut or miso helps.

• *Arrythmia.* In some cases calcium channel blockers cause rapid heartbeat and generalized palpitations. If you have a history of heart attack or stroke, be sure to mention this fact to your doctor before taking these drugs.

• *Edema (swelling of the extremities).* Approximately 10 percent of patients experience a swelling of the feet and ankles.

• *Flushing.* Flushing and an undue sensation of warmth occurs in about 25 percent of the people taking this type of medication.

• Other rare though possible reactions include dizziness, headache, blurred vision, and nervousness.

## 6. Centrally acting agents

*Profile.* Centrally acting agents are commonly prescribed to treat mild to moderate blood pressure. They are not usually used as a primary drug but are prescribed when more common antihypertensives like ACE inhibitors and beta-blockers prove ineffective. Centrally acting agents are also sometimes prescribed and taken along with a diuretic. Usually two to three weeks are necessary before blood pressure responds. *Warning:* Never abruptly discontinue a centrally acting antihypertensive. Work with your doctor to wean yourself off it slowly. Sudden withdrawl can precipitate serious and even fatal reactions.

*Mechanism of action.* Centrally acting agents behave exactly as their name implies, going directly to the central nervous system in the brain where blood pressure control originates. Here they bind to the brain cell receptors responsible for lowering the activity of the sympathetic nervous system, thus reducing blood pressure.

*Side effects.* Centrally acting agents can produce several troublesome side effects, which is one reason they are not commonly prescribed. These side effects include:

• *Drowsiness.* Perhaps the most common side effect of centrally acting agents, this drowsiness at times can become extreme, rendering a patient incapable of driving or performing complex motor activities on the job. Patients are also cautioned not to mix centrally acting agents with sedatives, tranquilizers, or antidepressant medications; the combination can severely impair functioning.

• *Dry mouth.* This is a relatively minor but for some people maddeningly irritating symptom that day and night seems never to go away. For some, chewing gum or sucking on slippery elm pills brings relief. Various over-the-counter preparations are also available to fight dry mouth. Ask at your local pharmacy.

• *Mild orthostatic hypotension.* A sudden drop in blood pressure resulting from standing up suddenly. (See the reference to orthostatic hypotension in the section on the alpha-blocker side effects, above.)

• *Raynaud's phenomenon.* A condition of reduced blood flow into the fingers and toes, causing tingling, discomfort, and a sense of numbing cold in the extremities.

## Medical Treatment versus Lifestyle Treatment

Every week new blood pressure drugs are being tested in laboratories throughout the world. As yet, no one has found the perfect antihypertensive, though many of the drugs described above are highly effective.

Should you take blood pressure medication?

It depends.

Generally speaking, all but the most conservative doctors are friendly toward the idea of trying to get your blood pressure down through natural means before prescribing a course of medication. Not all doctors think this way, but today many do. Perhaps most.

Of course, if you suffer from extremely high, stubborn hypertension, drug therapy is clearly the route to take. To allow such a condition to go untreated is folly indeed. At the same time, modifying your lifestyle with the methods and techniques explained in the chapters to come *while* on medication will produce many health-related benefits, in some cases reducing the need for drug therapy, or even making it unnecessary.

It's those in the gray areas whom this book primarily addresses: the men and women who never thought about their blood pressure when they were younger, but whose blood pressure is now creeping up year by year. It's for those who have a family history of hypertension, or a tendency in that direction; those whose poor lifestyle habits, such as improper diet, undue stress, being overweight, smoking, drinking, and lack of exercise are conducive to blood pressure extremes; those who are approaching the borderlines of elevated blood pressure, or who have already entered the mild to moderate zone.

It is these people who stand to gain the most from ordered lifestyle modifications.

Now that you have an overview of what high blood pressure is all about, your next step is to focus on the practical, hands-on, day-to-day techniques you can practice to control this condition naturally.

These techniques have worked for countless people. And they can work for you. It all boils down to establishing the proper living standards, and then sticking to them with a wholesome regularity. This means eating properly, resting properly, exercising properly, maintaining proper weight control, and protecting yourself against undue stress—in short, taking responsibility for your own state of health and treating your body as the precious receptacle of the mind and spirit that it is.

## PART II

# Controlling Your Blood Pressure Naturally: Three Proven Methods

# 3

# The Three-Step System to Natural Blood Pressure Control

## Where to Begin

In 1979 a national tabloid ran an interesting experiment. The newspaper asked a professor at Cornell University to design a questionnaire that tested people's knowledge of basic nutrition. The test was then administered to 120 physicians who were attending a conference of the American Medical Association.

The questionnaire asked a number of simple and straightforward questions, such as how much iron the average woman requires in her daily diet. The doctors were asked to pick the highest salt-containing foods from a list of common grocery items. They were asked to identify foods that contain the highest number of calories, and the lowest.

What was the result?

*Ninety percent of the physicians failed the test.*

In the years since this questionnaire was administered, American physicians' awareness of diet, weight control, and health-related lifestyle factors has clearly risen.

At the same time, conventional medicine remains

primarily drug-oriented in its approach; most doctors think of nutrition, prevention, and quality-of-life issues as secondary elements in the healing process. Clearly, if people are to supplement their physician-administered health care with quality-of-life enhancements, they must learn about—and implement—these enhancements on their own.

Where to begin?

As far as hypertension is concerned, at the beginning, with three of the most important nonpharmacological steps you can take to gain control of your blood pressure.

The steps are laid out in this chapter in a systematic and easy-to-follow format. None of them is difficult to put into practice, though all take commitment and stick-to-itiveness, especially at the beginning. Besides helping to manage blood pressure, moreover, a number of bonus effects come from following these steps. Make them part of your daily lifestyle and your state of health will gradually improve, your mental and emotional well-being will increase, and your longevity factor will be raised

What's more, this three-step plan incorporates a tried-and-true methodology. There is nothing magical about it. You can test its validity anytime you choose. Simply take your blood pressure on a regular basis. If the three-step plan works, that's wonderful! You'll no doubt wish to keep following it.

On the other hand, if the three-step plan (along with the dietary recommendations in the sections that follow) does not bring your blood pressure down after a reasonable amount of time, you've lost nothing in the trying. In fact, even if your blood pressure remains unchanged, other benefits will come from these efforts: you'll look better, you'll feel better, you'll be better.

It's a no-lose proposition.

## Begin at the Beginning

Here's the game plan:

A. Take your blood pressure right now, record it, then read through the following sections. Assimilate all the suggestions and information you can.

B. Put these suggestions into practice on a daily basis. Stick with them religiously.

C. Take your blood pressure after three weeks. Record the systolic and diastolic figures carefully. Some people keep a special notebook for the purpose.

D. Allow another three weeks to pass while you continue to follow the routine. Take your blood pressure again and record it. Then take it again three weeks later. Then again three weeks after that, for a total elapsed time of twelve weeks.

E. At the end of this three-month period, compare your first blood pressure reading with your last. Chances are you'll see a hefty improvement. Remember, even just a 2- or 5-point drop in the systolic reading and a 2- or 3-point drop in the diastolic can reduce your chances of cardiovascular disease. Count such reductions as a victory.

F. Continue following the plan. After six months, assess your progress again. Then again after a year.

With steady adherence to these methods your blood pressure should remain well under control for many years to come.

The three-step antihypertensive plan begins with weight control.

## Step One: Weight Control

### Weight Control and Hypertension

It is difficult to exaggerate the importance weight control plays in the management of high blood pressure. In many cases the loss of 10 or 20 extra pounds is enough to keep pressure problems in line. No medications are necessary.

Think about that.

Nothing else but weight control. No special diets. No daily trips to the gym. No medications or turning your life upside down. Just weight loss. This one critical step alone can prolong your life and perhaps even save it.

For this reason most health care professionals now agree that obesity is among the greatest risks for hypertension, an evaluation supported by the fact that at least 60 percent of Americans with high blood pressure are overweight.

Why is excess poundage conducive to high blood pressure?

No one understands the mechanism entirely, though theories abound.

Common sense, for instance, suggests that harboring too many unnecessary fat cells places an added load on the blood-pumping apparatus. This extra freight forces several of the major organs to work overtime, straining an already hard-working system. Like any other part of the body, fatty tissue requires a constant inflow of blood. Estimates have it that every pound of fat we add to our frames requires approximately a mile of capillaries to feed it. Think then of the pressure that an extra 20 or 30 pounds puts on a person's heart, lungs, and circulatory system.

Another theory claims that when we put on extra weight, the amount of insulin secreted by the pancreas increases proportionately. Insulin lowers the amount of sodium excreted through urination. This reduction increases fluid retention, a prime cause of hypertension.

Finally, it is also known that being seriously overweight increases a person's chances of acquiring a number of chronic and acute disorders. A sampling of the most significant ones includes:

- Type II diabetes
- intestinal obstruction
- heightened blood cholesterol levels
- heart attack
- cirrhosis of the liver
- cerebral hemorrhage
- kidney disease
- gout
- stroke
- gallbladder disease
- certain kinds of cancer

In a 1998 study published in the *Journal of the American Medical Association*, test subjects were helped to lose 8 to 10 pounds and to make certain dietary changes. At the end of two and a half years the researchers found that more than half the participants were less likely to have high blood pressure or to need blood pressure medication than those in the control group. As an added bonus, the subjects suffered fewer heart attacks and strokes.

An interesting point to note concerning the relationship between high blood pressure and being overweight is made by Kenneth H. Cooper, M.D., in his book *Overcoming Hypertension*. Dr. Cooper quotes several studies suggesting that *upper-body obesity*—that is, excess fat above the waistline and specifically in the abdomen and chest—is more likely to promote blood pressure problems than lower-body obesity, in the hips and thighs.

Dr. Cooper quotes a JAMA report in which the diastolic pressures of seventy-six middle-aged men all increased in direct proportion to the inches they added to their waist-to-hip girth ratio.

Another study of 227 patients—conducted in Cooper's own clinic—showed that among men aged thirty to fifty-nine, those carrying excess weight in the abdomen had higher blood pressures than men of comparable weight with large lower-body fat distribution. Researchers at Cooper's clinic concluded that hypertension is triggered not by a high proportion of body fat alone, but also by a high proportion of "body trunk largeness." For people experiencing an ever-expanding case of "middle-age bulge," this fact is of special significance.

We could go on for many pages quoting studies that demonstrate how perilous being overweight is for the health in general and blood pressure in particular. But you get the point; no doubt you've heard much of the same news already.

The question that comes up, of course, is whether or not everybody who is overweight has high blood pressure. "I'm ten pounds underweight," one woman remarked, "and my blood pressure is off the charts." "I'm forty pounds overweight," a man told us, "and my blood pressure is just fine."

The answer then is no, not every overweight person experiences an equivalent rise in blood pressure. But lots do—more than 50 percent. That's enough of a risk factor to make health care professionals rank weight control as a top priority for high blood pressure control, and equally important, as a fundamental method for preventing the condition in the first place.

The most important things to keep in mind about extra poundage and about the health of your circulatory system can be stated in three major caveats:

1. For many people, overweight and hypertension are related. If you are 10 or more pounds above your ideal weight, you are probably putting yourself at some degree of risk.
2. Lose weight and you'll most likely see a reduction in your blood pressure. No guarantees, but the odds are strongly on your side.
3. Keep the extra weight off and your blood pressure will probably remain low as well. Put it back on and your blood pressure will probably rise.

**Finding Your Ideal Weight**

How overweight are people in the United States?

A study carried out at the National Center for Health Statistics in the Centers for Disease Control and Prevention revealed that approximately *55 percent of all Americans* weigh too much in relation to their size and build. This percentage, the Center discovered, has increased by almost a *third* since the early 1980s, and it appears to be on the climb despite Americans' increased awareness of the value of lean, no-fat eating.

How much weight is overweight?

The short answer is that people who are 20 to 30 percent over their ideal body weight—more on ideal body weight below—are carrying too many pounds.

The long, more complex answer is based on the relationship between the amount of fatty tissue that a man or woman has and the amount of nonfatty tissue.

Precise clinical standards for this measurement are by no means unanimous, and recommendations for an "acceptable" ratio of fatty tissue to total body weight tend to vary. For men, a range of from 12 to 25 percent body fat is considered acceptable. For women, 18 to 30 percent body fat is within the realm of ideal weight.

How does one determine the percentage of body fat?

There are several methods, all of which require a health care professional's assistance.

The use of skinfold calipers, for example, targets the layers of skin in key areas of the body, using the thickness of these layers to determine overall body fat readings. Another system, bioelectrical impedance analysis (BIA), uses electrical resistance to measure fat cell ratio. Underwater weighing, probably the most accurate of all methods but also the most expensive and elaborate, requires special tanks and weighing equipment.

If all the above methods for determining ideal weight seem too complex, you can simply use an insurance company ideal weight chart. While the figures on these charts differ slightly from company to company (and from year to year), the calculations, based on a person's height and build, are all more or less in the same ballpark.

Table 1 below shows a representative ideal weight chart from Met Life. Check the figures against your own height and build, keeping in mind that 20 to 30 percent over ideal weight qualifies as overweight.

### Table 1: Ideal Weight*

MALES

| Height Feet | Inches | Small build | Medium build | Large build |
|---|---|---|---|---|
| 5 | 2 | 128–134 | 131–141 | 138–150 |
| 5 | 3 | 130–136 | 133–143 | 140–153 |
| 5 | 4 | 132–138 | 135–145 | 142–156 |
| 5 | 5 | 134–140 | 137–148 | 144–160 |
| 5 | 6 | 136–142 | 139–151 | 146–164 |
| 5 | 7 | 138–145 | 142–154 | 149–168 |
| 5 | 8 | 140–148 | 145–157 | 152–172 |
| 5 | 9 | 142–151 | 148–160 | 155–176 |
| 5 | 10 | 144–154 | 151–163 | 158–180 |
| 5 | 11 | 146–157 | 154–166 | 161–184 |
| 6 | 0 | 149–160 | 157–170 | 164–188 |
| 6 | 1 | 152–164 | 160–174 | 168–192 |
| 6 | 2 | 155–168 | 164–178 | 172–197 |
| 6 | 3 | 158–172 | 167–182 | 172–202 |
| 6 | 4 | 162–176 | 171–187 | 181–207 |

## Table 1: Ideal Weight* continued

FEMALES

| Height Feet | Inches | Small build | Medium build | Large build |
|---|---|---|---|---|
| 4 | 10 | 102–111 | 109–121 | 118–131 |
| 4 | 11 | 103–113 | 111–123 | 120–134 |
| 5 | 0 | 104–115 | 113–126 | 122–137 |
| 5 | 1 | 106–118 | 115–129 | 125–140 |
| 5 | 2 | 108–121 | 118–132 | 128–143 |
| 5 | 3 | 111–124 | 121–135 | 131–147 |
| 5 | 4 | 114–127 | 124–138 | 134–151 |
| 5 | 5 | 117–130 | 127–141 | 137–155 |
| 5 | 6 | 120–133 | 130–144 | 140–159 |
| 5 | 7 | 123–136 | 133–147 | 143–163 |
| 5 | 8 | 126–139 | 136–150 | 146–167 |
| 5 | 9 | 129–142 | 139–153 | 149–170 |
| 5 | 10 | 132–145 | 142–156 | 152–173 |
| 5 | 11 | 135–148 | 145–159 | 155–176 |
| 6 | 0 | 138–151 | 148–162 | 158–179 |

*Based on information from Metropolitan Life Insurance Company Health and Safety Education Division

Finally, if none of the above methods suits your needs, there is an easier way still of determining your ideal weight. A rule of thumb that gives a conservative but workable figure is as follows:

*For women:* Given a height of five feet, assume an ideal weight of 100 pounds. Add 5 pounds for every inch above this height. For example, if you are five foot one, your ideal weight is somewhere in the area of 105 pounds. If you are five foot two, your ideal weight is around 110.

*For men:* Given a height of five feet, assume an ideal weight of 106 pounds. Add 6 pounds for every inch above this height. For example, if you are five foot one, your ideal weight is in the area of 112 pounds. If five foot two, your ideal weight is around 118 pounds.

As mentioned, this is a conservative measurement technique and assumes a rather slight figure. If your bone structure is of medium size, add another 5 pounds to your ideal weight estimate. If you are stocky, add 10 pounds.

## The Science and Art of Losing Weight: Tricks, Tactics, and Techniques

Once you've calculated your ideal weight and determined how many pounds you must shed to reach that target (or at least approach its vicinity), the process of slimming down begins in earnest—the famous "Battle of the Bulge."

As you no doubt know, a vast number of weight-loss diets, many of them gratifyingly effective, are available today in books and magazines. For simply staying trim, as well as for keeping hypertension under control, the recipes featured in the final section of this book are excellent as well.

The challenge to losing pounds, however, is not in finding a good diet. Good diets abound. The real challenges are:

• feeling motivated enough to adopt a new eating style,

• developing habits and attitudes that support this new diet (including physical aids like exercise and mental aids like motivational planning),

• sticking to the new eating plan long enough to lose the desired number of pounds,

• keeping the weight off once you've achieved a desirable weight.

The following tricks, tactics, and techniques are all

designed to help you accomplish these goals. Wise dieting, as any weight-loss veteran knows, is not simply based on the food you eat. It's also based on how, when, where, what, and why you eat.

To guide you through this maze there are numerous tricks of the dieting trade, a number of which are featured below. Just remember: Weight loss is not simply an eating thing. It's a lifestyle thing, an attitude and environment thing as well as a menu. Which means that the best way to lose pounds effectively is to surround yourself with the kinds of personal helps and supports that make your task as easy as possible. Some of the best of these are:

**1. Stay focused, stay enthusiastic, and stay committed**

Experts agree: The most important device you can have in a toolbox of dieting strategies is a can-do attitude.

What does this mean, exactly?

It means that if you are attempting to lose weight you must *want* to lose weight. More important, you must want to lose weight for your own sake, not for the sake of others.

Attitude is everything. Study after study has demonstrated that when a challenge presents itself, a person's success rate rises or falls on his or her degree of commitment. People who attempt to quit smoking, innumerable studies show, do best when they quit for themselves and not for spouses, children, or concerned friends. People who struggle with addictions such as gambling or drugs overcome them most frequently when they are strongly self-motivated.

The same is true for weight loss. To get the job done quickly and effectively, it's essential that you diet out of a sense of personal need and conviction, not because your doctor has advised it, or your loved ones urge it.

Where does the sense of conviction come from?

It is generated by three impulses:

1. a desire to improve and maintain your physical health, and specifically to control your hypertension, prevent the onslaught of cardiovascular disease, and maximize your life span;
2. a desire to slim down and look your physical best;
3. a desire to feel good mentally—to be more confident, have more self-esteem, and experience all-round feelings of accomplishment, fulfillment, and self-satisfaction.

Three excellent reasons, and three powerful motivators: better health, improved body image, and an increased sense of mental and emotional well-being. Strive to keep these three factors in mind when approaching your diet and the rest will take care of itself.

### 2. Old Faithful: simply count your calories

There are, as mentioned, innumerable weight-loss diets available today, many of them ingenious, and some of them effective. The problem in choosing which of these plans to follow is that the options are overwhelming and the diets dauntingly complex. As one man who was dieting to control his hypertension remarked to me, "You have to be a rocket scientist to figure out all the measurements, substitutions, and cross-portions you eat every time you sit down to my new diet."

If you find yourself boggled by too many choices and confused by the elaborate dos and don'ts of various weight-loss programs, your best bet may be to return to basics and lose weight the old-fashioned way: by counting calories.

There are several advantages to this method, the major one being its simplicity.

Here's the basic equation: If you ingest more calories than your body needs each day, these extra calories are converted into fat. Presto! You put on weight. If you take in fewer calories than your body needs each day, surplus fat cells are burned away. Presto! You lose weight.

That's about all there is to it.

What is a calorie? To a physicist, a calorie is the amount of heat necessary to raise one gram of water to a temperature of 1°C. For nutritional purposes, a calorie is the fundamental unit of energy contained in any food. A teaspoonful of butter, for example, contains 45 calories—45 units of nutritional energy. A half cup of blueberries contains the same amount.

While the number of calories a person requires every day to maintain optimum health varies according to his or her physical makeup (factors include physical size, sex, age, level of daily activity, and metabolism), there are several rules of thumb that can be applied. One of the best is as follows:

If you are an active person involved in a nonsedentary profession, multiply your present weight by 16.

The resulting figure shows how many calories you need each day to maintain your present weight. For example, if you weigh 150 pounds, you will need 2,400 calories a day to keep your weight at status quo.

If you are an inactive person who works at a sedentary job, multiply your present weight by 14. The resulting figure shows how many calories you need each day to maintain your present weight. For example, if you weigh 150 pounds, you need 2,100 calories a day to remain at status quo.

How do you use the calorie-counting method for weight loss?

Simply reduce your normal daily intake of calories by 500 to 1,000 calories a day.

This means that if you require 2,500 calories a day to maintain your present weight, you can cut the number to 1,500 to 2,000 calories a day. If you require 2,300 a day, reduce this figure to 1,300 to 1,800.

How many calories can you safely eliminate from your diet?

In general, it's a good idea not to eliminate more than 1,000 calories a day from your regular food intake, and never to reduce overall caloric intake below 1,200 a day. Anything below this level leaves people so hungry and frustrated they usually give up their dieting ambitions within a week.

An important related factor in this equation is your daily degree of activity.

If, for instance, you are a highly active person who weighs 150 pounds, you will lose weight if you cut your regular 2,400 calories to 1,900, a reduction of 500 calories a day. If you are inactive you will need to cut more, say from 2,400 calories to 1600, a reduction of 800 calories a day. Each person has his or her own needs and must determine optimal calorie intake on the basis of activity level and body type. Exercise, it should be added, will help the whole process along very nicely. More on this in the next section.

How many pounds a week can one lose by counting calories?

It depends on the individual. A pound a week is typical with a 500-a-day calorie reduction, though some people, especially active types, lose up to two pounds. More than this is too abrupt a shock for the body and is not recommended.

How does one measure the number of calories in any given food?

Calorie charts and calorie counters are available at any bookstore or supermarket. Find a pocket-sized edition and keep it with you. (Most calorie-counting booklets are small and portable.) Then, when preparing food or ordering it in a restaurant, consult your calorie counter. Add up the approximate caloric value of the foods you are about to eat, making sure that your three daily meals stay within the 500-calorie-reduction limit. After a while you'll become familiar with the calorie count of the foods you eat most often, and you'll find it less necessary to consult the booklet.

To get you started in the adventure of calorie counting, Table 2 profiles the calorie count in a number of common foods.

## Table 2: Calories in Common Foods

| Food | Amount | Calorie count |
| --- | --- | --- |
| **Breads** | | |
| Bread, white | 1 slice | 75 |
| Bread, whole wheat | 1 slice | 60 |
| Hamburger roll | 1 | 120 |
| Muffin | 1 (3″ diameter) | 120 |
| Roll, Parker House | 1 | 160 |
| **Cakes and cookies** | | |
| Apple pie | 1 slice | 300 |
| Chocolate cake with icing | 1 slice | 250 |
| Chocolate chip cookie | 1 (3″ diameter) | 100 |
| Doughnut | 1 (3½″ diameter) | 180 |
| Pound cake | 1 slice | 150 |
| **Cereals** | | |
| Cornflakes | 1 cup | 115 |
| Oatmeal | 1 cup | 120 |
| Puffed wheat | 1 cup | 60 |
| **Dairy products** | | |
| Butter | 1″ pat | 35 |
| Cheese, American | 1 ounce | 100 |
| Cheese, Brie | 1 ounce | 120 |
| Cheese, cottage, whole-milk | 1 cup | 260 |
| Cream, half-and-half | 2 tablespoons | 40 |
| Milk, skim | 1 cup | 90 |
| Milk, whole | 1 cup | 160 |

| Food | Amount | Calorie count |
|---|---|---|
| **Fruits** | | |
| Apple | 1 (2½″ diameter) | 85 |
| Avocado | 5 ounces | 185 |
| Banana | 1 (7″ fruit) | 80 |
| Cherries | ½ cup | 40 |
| Grapefruit | ½ (3½″ fruit) | 40 |
| Orange | 1 (3″ fruit) | 80 |
| Pear | 1 cup sliced | 60 |
| Raisins | ½ cup | 240 |
| Strawberries | ½ cup | 150 |
| Watermelon | 1 slice (2 pounds) | 110 |
| **Meats and poultry** | | |
| Beef, hamburger | 3 ounces | 200 |
| Beef, pot roast | 3 ounces | 250 |
| Beef, slice | 3 ounces | 250 |
| Chicken, broiled | ¼ small broiler | 115 |
| Chicken, fried | ½ breast | 150 |
| Lamb, loin chop | 3 ounces | 300 |
| Lamb, roast leg of | 3 ounces | 230 |
| Pork, bacon | 1 slice | 30 |
| Pork, chop | 3 ounces | 330 |
| Pork, ham, cured | 3 ounces | 250 |
| Pork, sausage links | 2 (4″ links) | 125 |
| Turkey, dark meat | 3 ounces | 145 |
| Turkey, light meat | 3 ounces | 175 |
| Veal, cutlet | 3 ounces | 200 |
| **Fish and seafood** | | |
| Bass, fresh | 1 pound | 752 |
| Clams, steamed | 1 pound | 230 |
| Cod, fresh | 1 pound | 711 |
| Flounder, fresh | 1 pound | 900 |
| Haddock, fresh | 1 pound | 765 |
| Herring, pickled | 1 pound | 995 |

| Food | Amount | Calorie count |
| --- | --- | --- |
| Lobster, steamed | 1 medium-sized | 190 |
| Oysters, fresh | 1 cup | 578 |
| Perch, fresh | 1 pound | 430 |
| Red snapper, fresh | 1 pound | 410 |
| Salmon, canned | 1 pound | 652 |
| Salmon, fresh | 1 pound | 830 |
| Salmon, smoked | 1 pound | 802 |
| Sardines | 1 pound | 1,511 |
| Shad, fresh | 1 pound | 843 |
| Shrimp, fresh | 1 pound | 1,001 |
| Swordfish, fresh | 1 pound | 749 |
| Trout, fresh | 1 pound | 901 |
| Tuna, canned in oil | 1 pound | 874 |
| Tuna, canned in water | 1 pound | 417 |
| **Nuts** | | |
| Almonds | 10–12 | 70 |
| Cashews | 10–12 | 100 |
| Peanuts | 2 tablespoons | 100 |
| Peanut butter, crunchy | 1 tablespoon | 105 |
| Pecans | 10 large | 100 |
| Walnuts | 2 tablespoons | 100 |
| **Vegetables** | | |
| Broccoli | ½ cup | 25 |
| Carrot | ½ cup | 25 |
| Corn, on the cob | 1 ear (6″) | 90 |
| Corn, kernels | ½ cup | 75 |
| Peas | ½ cup | 65 |
| Potato, baked | 1 (2½″ long) | 150 |
| Potato chips | 10 | 100 |
| Potato, mashed | ½ cup | 75 |
| Squash | ½ cup | 20 |
| Tomatoes | ½ cup | 35 |

A final caution related to calories. You've heard it said many times, no doubt, but it's important enough to repeat: Besides causing weight to skyrocket, high-fat foods such as fatty meats, most junk foods, and dairy products (especially butter, cream, and whole milk) are intensely cholesterol-heavy, and should be kept to a minimum in any antihypertensive diet. We'll have a good deal more to say on the subject in the dietary chapters ahead.

### 3. Exercise

An accumulating body of evidence suggests that people who accompany their weight-loss program with a regular regimen of daily exercise lose weight faster than those who do not exercise. They lose this weight in the right places (i.e., the abdomen, buttocks, and thighs) and keep it off longer than those who perform little or no physical activity.

There are a number of reasons why this is so.

Exercise supplements the benefits of dieting, burning up calories and consuming nutrients that would otherwise be deposited as excess pounds. One of the difficulties that dieters encounter with low-calorie diets is that their resting metabolic rates decrease along with the lower number of calories consumed. Several studies demonstrate that this trend is reversed by daily exercise, which speeds up metabolism and hence the process of fat burning.

It is likewise known that vigorous exercise practiced at least four times a week releases chemicals into the blood that slow down the transmission of hunger signals to the brain and that increase the flow of blood to the stomach, generating feelings of fullness and satiation. While popular wisdom has it that exercise burns energy and increases the need for food, the truth is that exercise is an appetite suppressant.

A vigorous exercise program also affects the distribution of adipose tissue throughout the body. Hypertensive patients with an excess of fat stored above the hips, as we have seen, tend to develop cardiovascular problems more frequently than patients whose weight is the same but whose fat is below belt level. Exercise, especially aerobic exercise, helps redistribute weight more evenly, reducing the dangerous abdominal fat that is so closely associated with heart and circulation problems.

Note finally that exercise is a mood elevator. A robust round of physical activity increases the opioid peptides in the bloodstream that are partly responsible for generating feelings of happiness and gratification. The resulting sense of well-being makes us feel good about ourselves, and this in turn stimulates our motivation to slim down and get in shape.

Exercise and weight-reduction programs, in other words, are complementary self-help aids that should be thought of as the dieter's one-two punch. When paired they generate far more effective results than when practiced alone. Table 3 shows the caloric weight-loss averages generated by selected sports and work activities.

### Table 3: Calorie-Burning Activities

| Activity or exercise | Calories expended per hour (approximate) |
| --- | --- |
| **Sports** | |
| Bicycle riding | 450 |
| Calisthenics | 300 |
| Golf | 250 |
| Jogging | 600 |
| Racquetball | 600 |
| Rollerblading | 375 |
| Tennis | 400 |
| Walking | 450 |
| **Work activities** | |
| Cleaning house | 200 |
| Climbing stairs | 600 |
| Mowing the lawn | 250 |
| Sawing wood | 500 |
| Vacuuming | 250 |
| Washing floors | 350 |

## 4. Make haste slowly: six important points to observe when dieting

As an old saying has it, "What takes a long time to come stays a long time as well."

Nowhere is this saying more apt than in the matter of dieting. Crash diets have their place, perhaps, especially if a person is slimming down for appearance's sake. But for hypertensives who are attempting to rethink their lifestyles and redesign their lives according to moderate, commonsense health ideals, the day-to-day, step-at-a-time approach is the most sensible *and* the safest.

First, follow a diet that suits your personal needs. Don't be taken in by the fantastic claims you hear about the latest fad diet. If these claims seem too good to be true, they probably are. The best recommendation is word of mouth. Talk to friends. Ask around. See what plans successful dieters use. Look for a weight-loss program that meshes with your lifestyle. Try it out. If it doesn't work as well as expected, try another. Speed is not a priority here. As far as dieting goes, you have the right to take your time.

Second, establish realistic weight-loss goals and stick to them. One or 2 pounds a week, or 6 to 8 pounds a month, is a reasonable aim. Anything more than this can get you into trouble. Studies of weight-loss psychology show that many dieters establish impossible target weights for themselves. When they fall short of these goals they become discouraged and give up. Losing weight in slow but steady increments has the reverse effect, motivating dieters with a number of small daily victories. As far as the weight-loss game goes, nothing succeeds like steady, day-by-day success.

Third, start your diet at the right time. If you are under a great deal of stress right now, if things are in a period of flux, if there is a major crisis or a major change taking place, you don't need the extra pressure of a diet to complicate life. Hold off until the smoke clears. Then, when your life is back on an even keel, go for it. Studies have shown that people who begin dieting in an untroubled state of mind tend to succeed more than those who are worried and depressed.

Fourth, establish a dieting home environment that works for you. Identify the specific foods and eating habits that get you into trouble. ("What the eye doesn't see," goes a Chinese proverb, "the heart doesn't yearn for.") Do you have a quart of ice cream in the fridge, for example? Is there a bread basket on the table? Determine which temptations trigger your hunger for forbidden foods. Then eliminate them from the table, shelf, and refrigerator. That's for starters. Also consider: When's the time of day you tend to eat most lavishly? Between meals? Midnight munching? Identify the hours you're most likely to slip, then make sure you have a stock of nonfattening snacks on hand. Finally, there are the social cues. If you tend to eat especially fattening foods at restaurants, curtail your dining-out activities for a while. If family meals are a problem, talk to the cook and have another family member monitor your portions. Pay attention to these and similar situational cues and you'll find that you've done part of the dieting work simply by avoiding temptation.

Fifth, realize that you will inevitably experience plateaus, periods of time in which no matter how hard you try to lose weight your body won't oblige. When this occurs, don't lose heart. It's all part of the weight-loss process. A good trick for getting past these times is to increase your daily exercise and physical activity. Just know in advance that the plateaus are going to come. They happen to everyone. But know too that they will pass, and that they will be followed by periods of rapid and gratifying weight loss.

Sixth, be gentle with yourself. Now and then you're going to give in to those cravings for ice cream and buttered croissants. At least, most people do. If you're one of those with an iron will, that's great; this advice is not for you. But if you're human like the rest of us, chances are you'll slip and slip and slip again on the slopes of Mount Diet. When you do, don't beat yourself up for it. Guilt and self-chastisement are not only pointless, they are self-demoralizing, and ultimately they cause you to lose heart. When you slip in the midst of your diet simply tell yourself you'll do better tomorrow. Then try again. In the dieting game, step by step takes you a long way.

## 5. Take advantage of dieting's many tricks

There are innumerable tricks of the dieting game, many of which really help. Here's a sampling:

• Before every meal drink one or two glasses of water. Your appetite is ruled by your stomach. If your stomach is partially filled you'll eat less. Try this one. It really works.

• Make small portions seem larger. Pad the chicken pieces with lots of lettuce. Add sprouts, celery, and tomatoes to the main course. When preparing and arranging foods, concentrate on making low-calorie foods appear especially delicious and tempting.

• The minute you begin to feel full, stop eating. Overeating is a principal cause of overweight. So pace yourself. And remember, even if you feel slightly hungry when you leave the table, that feeling of being full will come in a few minutes, after all the food has reached your stomach and begins to digest.

• Eat slowly. Savor the food. Allow yourself to become conscious of the texture of what you're eating and of the many subtle tastes that we ordinarily miss. Eating a meal slowly fills us up sooner. And by savoring the food along the way we heighten our enjoyment.

• Drink a cup of fat-free buttermilk in the afternoon before lunch and in the evening before dinner. It will fill you up, nourish you, and cut down on the amount of food you're likely to eat at those meals.

• Have your largest meal in the middle of the day, when your digestion is still vigorous (it slows down at night), and then eat a light supper. Many people lose weight using this trick alone. Some people go it one further, having their largest meal at breakfast and their smallest meal at night, following the dictum "Eat breakfast like a king, lunch like a citizen, dinner like a pauper."

• Record your progress. Then reward yourself as you go along. Some people write down their daily weight in a log or notebook. When they lose a pound or three they reward themselves with a new dress, a CD, a pleasant night out with friends. Educators have long known that people learn better if they are rewarded for their successes rather than punished for their failures.

• Read labels when shopping. Many "low-fat" and "lite" foods offer less reduction in fat, calories, and cholesterol than you may think. Standards in this area are regulated by law, so carefully check all the labels before purchasing food.

• For those sudden cravings, a fat-based food often satisfies hunger pangs more effectively than the food most of us reach for when we're hungry—sugar. If you're feeling appetite pangs, try a piece of bread with a thin smear of butter on it. Eat a salad with an olive oil and vinegar dressing. Enjoy a tablespoonful of crunchy natural-style peanut butter. Such small amounts of high-quality fats are not going to hurt, and you'll be surprised at how well and quickly they stem the appetite.

• Crisp, crunchy snacks are solid aids. They fill us up and at the same time give us plenty of chewing action, a process that mysteriously helps gratify food cravings. Celery is effective in this department, as are carrots, firm fruits like apples, and also red peppers, green peppers, radishes, sunflower seeds, and cabbage.

• Also look for low-fat and nonfat foods with a smooth, creamy consistency. Use nonfat plain yogurt as a base for dips, or puree it with fruit as a dessert. Nonfat buttermilk with spices and fruit makes an excellent shake.

• Finally, remember this: The hardest part of creative snacking is to reach for those low-fat, low-calorie foods first. Once you have them in your hand and in your mouth, you've won half the battle.

## Step Two: Exercise

### The Real Scoop on Exercise and Hypertension

Aerobic exercise is a major antirisk factor in reducing hypertension and a powerful nonpharmachological aid. If practiced three or four times a week over an extended period of time, it exerts measurable positive effects on blood pressure in a large number of patients. Many people see tangible benefits within a month or two.

What's more, regular physical exercise not only curtails pressure rates but produces generous side benefits that include enhanced cardiovascular health, reduced feelings of stress and fatigue, improvement in physical appearance, and a global sense of mental tranquillity and emotional well-being.

What's the downside?

None, really. Except for a few rare exceptions that we'll talk about below. Otherwise exercise is a no-lose proposition.

Since the 1930s, when doctors began to notice that professional athletes consistently display lower blood pressures than their sedentary peers, numerous studies have been made to determine the relationship between exercise and blood pressure. The results have provided strong evidence that blood pressure and exercise are linked, and that an organized regimen of bicycling, aerobic exercise, swimming, fast walking, dancing, or one of many other exercises produces valuable health benefits. These include:

• A possible drop of from 10 to 20 mm Hg in the systolic blood pressure, and from 2 to 10 in the diastolic. Results vary from person to person. But in a majority of cases regular exercise tends to lower readings.

• A lowered risk of stroke and heart attack. A number of long-term epidemiologic studies support this finding.

• Help for people who are trying to stop smoking. Researchers believe that the positive psychological effects of exercise, with their concomitant improvement in self-image and relief from stress, help give smokers the resolve they need to quit.

• Lowered risk of osteoporosis. Regular exercise helps delay the loss of calcium from the bones and makes the bones more resistant to fracture. In 1984 the National Institutes of Health Consensus Development Panel recommended a course of "modest weight-bearing exercise" as a possible preventive measure against osteoporosis.

• A possible reduction in the risk of atherosclerosis.

• Relief from stress, fatigue, chronic anxiety, and depression. A meta-analysis of thirty-four clinical studies done to determine the relationship between exercise and stress showed that aerobically fit individuals had a substantially reduced stress response compared with those in the control groups.

• An increase in "good" serum high-density lipoprotein (HDL) cholesterol levels, and a reduction in serum triglycerides and possibly in low-density lipoprotein (LDL) levels.

• Control over certain forms of diabetes. In some cases exercise increases glucose utilization and lowers the need for insulin.

• Help keeping the body trim and supple. Improvement in muscle tone. Control over body weight and maintenance of a better muscle-to-fat ratio. Improves both perceived body image and actual physical appearance.

• Slowing down of the aging process, along with a possible increase in longevity. As we age, our oxygen consumption is reduced at a rate of approximately 1 percent per year. Exercise slows this decline.

Quite a list of benefits. And there's more.

As far as hypertension and the human circulatory

apparatus are concerned, aerobic workouts keep blood vessels elastic and flexible. They reduce the incidence of vein constriction with its consequent threat of hypertension, and they help stave off age-related hardening of the arteries.

A study at the National Institute on Aging's Gerontology Research Center in Baltimore shows that a regular program of aerobic fitness training can delay age-associated arterial stiffness, especially among the aging. Members of the study's research team recruited fourteen robust older males aged fifty-four to seventy-five who jogged on an average of thirty miles a week. Studying these senior athletes, researchers found they had approximately 30 percent less vessel stiffness than their sedentary contemporaries.

Dozens of other studies confirm these and related findings.

For example, according to one report in the journal *Hypertension*, twelve hypertensive men were given a ten- to twenty-week aerobic workout program. After ten weeks, a reduction of 20 mm Hg systolic and 10 mm Hg diastolic pressure was noted among 50 percent of the patients.

During a study at the San Diego State College Exercise Laboratory, twenty-three men with an average blood pressure of 159/105 were put on a one-hour-a-day exercise program consisting of a half hour of calisthenics and a half hour of walking or jogging. After six months, the mean blood pressure of the group dropped to 146/93.

A similar study conducted by Dr. David Siscovic at

the University of North Carolina determined that men who exercise 140 minutes a week have 60 percent less chance of dying from cardiac and circulatory disease than men of the same age who do not exercise on a regular basis.

At the University of Pennsylvania, the health of 7,685 male graduates was studied for several decades. Many physiological variables were taken into consideration. At the end of the study, subjects who participated in sports or exercise programs were approximately half as likely to develop hypertension than those who did not.

Thus, while there are doubters and qualifiers here and there among members of the medical profession, generally speaking the verdict is in on exercise and hypertension. This verdict is based on the results of numerous clinical studies plus the experience of thousands of health care professionals and millions of exercisers. Its message is clear and strong: *Exercise works.* Do it, the message says, and the odds are that your hypertension will improve. In certain cases it may vanish completely.

What further reasons do any of us need to begin?

## Which Kind of Exercise Is Best for Blood Pressure Control?

There are three types of physical exercise:

- isotonic
- isometric
- isokinetic

Here's a profile of each:

*Isotonic exercise,* also known as *aerobic* or *dynamic exercise*, involves the vigorous use of large muscle systems (especially the arms, legs, and breathing apparatus) in any activity involving prolonged and low-resistance motion. During aerobic exercise the heart rate is raised dramatically and remains elevated for sustained periods of time. The heart-lung system is stimulated and circulation quickens. Oxygen intake goes up and increased amounts of blood shift into the muscles. The elimination of waste products is speeded up through sweating and loss of body fluids. Frequent performance of isotonic exercise raises endurance as well as overall functioning.

Examples of isotonics include fast walking, jogging, dancing, aerobic exercise, swimming, tennis, cycling, using a treadmill, cross-country skiing—any continuous activity that raises the heartbeat and produces vigorous body movement.

*Isometric* or *static exercise* takes place when the muscles of the body are tensed and contracted, usually while straining against a fixed point of resistance. Lifting weights is a classic example. Isometrics provide little or no aerobic workout, and as a general rule they do little to improve cardiovascular endurance.

Anatomically, there is a minimum of joint movement during isometric exercise. The heart and lungs remain relatively unstimulated, while the muscles increase in tension but do not undergo an appreciable extension in length. Isometric exercise is especially beneficial for toning and sculpting specific groups of muscles. It increases physical strength and aids in body-building development.

*Isokinetic exercise* is a relatively new fitness category that combines elements of both isometric and isotonic exercise. Isokinetics develop muscle strength and stimulate the cardiovascular system by means of both pushing against resistance (isometric) and exercising the large muscle groups in a sustained, heartbeat-raising activity (isotonic). Exercise bicycles, rowing machines, and stair-climbing machines offer versions of isokinetic exercise.

Which form of exercise is best for combating hypertension?

Isometric exercises tend to involve concerted bursts of activity followed by periods of inactivity. Think of a weight lifter snatching 200 pounds in one excruciating swoop, then placing the weights down and resting between lifts. These sudden adrenaline explosions shoot the blood pressure up, then drop it abruptly. Such fluctuations are well tolerated by highly trained athletes. But for those on the borders of high blood pressure, such on-off expenditures do little over the long term to improve blood pressure, and in the short term they can be dangerous. Isometric exercise is thus usually counterindicated for anyone concerned with controlling hypertension.

Better for our purposes are isotonic/aerobic and isokinetic exercise. The following section contains an exercise honor role featuring a quality-graded selection of the physical activities most recommended for controlling and preventing high blood pressure.

## Swimming

In many people's estimation swimming is the best aerobic workout the body can enjoy. In swimming, unlike jogging and action sports, the torso is suspended in water, and this protects against pounding pressure on the joints. Yet water also provides a natural force of resistance for the entire axial skeleton to push against. All the major muscle groups work in sync, elevating the heart rate without pushing it to sudden extremes, and putting the entire system through a rigorous, full-body workout. In comparable time and distance, a person paddling in a pool or lake burns 25 percent more calories than a jogger. Swimmers thus receive all the benefits of a full-body aerobic workout without experiencing the damaging side effects that more demanding sports bring.

To receive full benefit, you should swim for thirty to forty-five minutes three or four times a week. Swimming laps at a moderate pace is the most systematic form of workout, though water exercises, treading water, and even a sustained dog paddle all have their benefits.

## Bicycling

Peddling a bike is another superior way of staying fit and at the same time receiving the full benefits of an aerobic workout. Unless you push too hard—and this is true in any exercise—cycling is safe, especially if you work up to it slowly, cycling a few miles a day in the beginning, then adding to your time and distance at a moderate pace.

Cycling mainly exercises the lower extremities, though the entire body benefits, especially the heart and lungs. Just try peddling up a hill for ten minutes at a time, and your lungs and heart rate will agree.

If you intend to practice outdoor bike riding, begin with a half hour of moderate cycling three or four times a week, being sure to go easy on the hills. After the first week, add five minutes to your cycling time, then five more minutes each week for several months. At the end of this time your fitness level will be way up the scale. You can then determine how many minutes a week you wish to cycle, and how difficult a course you choose to ride.

If you are working indoors on a cycling machine, half an hour of moderate peddling four times a week is a good pace to set in the beginning. As the weeks pass you can extend your cycling time to forty-five minutes a day three or four times a week, then to an hour. You may wish to gradually ratchet up the resistance level on the machine as your legs become stronger, and as your desire for a more rigorous workout increases.

### Walking

The number of benefits that accrue from walking are just beginning to be appreciated by medical professionals. Though jogging was the aerobic exercise of choice during the 1970s and 1980s, it has gradually become clear that walking provides almost as effective a cardiovascular workout without the joint-pounding that jogging brings.

Like running, walking conditions all the major muscle groups, including those in the arms if the arms are swung purposefully with each stride. Walking increases circulation, builds endurance, improves posture and body alignment, and elevates mood. It is a highly enjoyable social activity if practiced with a friend or relative in agreeable surroundings.

The benefits of walking for the health of your blood pressure can be maximized by following these guidelines:

1. Maintain proper posture while you walk. Keep your ears aligned over your shoulders and your shoulders aligned over your hips. Let your arms swing freely. Pump them while you walk if you wish, for greater oxygen intake. Be careful of leaning, jutting your chin, swaying from side to side, or "falling" forward as you walk. A good trick is to imagine that there is an invisible thread attached to the top of your head. As you walk the thread pulls you upward, serving as a reference point for balance and straightness.

2. Avoid tensing your shoulders, back, and face. Ease your shoulders, let your arms swing freely, keep your stomach and chest loose and open. No pressure or strife. Just relax and enjoy the day.

3. Breathe deeply as you stride. Shallow breathing deprives you of the full benefits of walking. Concentrate on taking full, deep breaths. Let them start from the bottom of your stomach and move upward into the middle and upper parts of your lungs. Walking, by its very nature, is an aerobic exercise—it brings oxygen

into the body. Maximize this benefit with vigorous breathing.

4.  Maintain a positive attitude while you walk. Now is *not* the time for thinking about the mortgage. Make your walking hour a private time of escape from personal problems. Allow yourself a stress-free period of the day. Look forward to it. Make walking a pleasant, joyful activity.

If you are just starting on a regimen of walking, forty-five minutes a day performed at a brisk clip three or four times a week is adequate. As the weeks pass and as your legs and cardiovascular functions strengthen, you will want to increase both speed and distance. Walking three miles a day every day is one of the best and safest aerobic workouts available to exercisers, especially for people over forty. Take advantage of it.

**AEROBIC ACTIVITIES: THE B LIST**

## Jogging

While jogging is certainly an exemplary aerobic exercise, and while the euphoria a three- or four-mile jog generates can be exhilarating, there are enough problems connected with this pastime to relegate it to the B list.

First, running pounds and punishes the joints. Hips and knees suffer especially. The effects of this daily beating may not be apparent right away. But over the months, over the years, the punishment takes its toll. The origins of ankle and knee degeneration that appear at midlife can often be traced to years of hard pounding on a runner's course. Among those who take up running at a later age, especially people who have been sedentary for most of their lives, jogging is known to trigger a host of orthopedic ailments, including tendon injuries, stress fractures of the bones, and aggravated arthritis.

Second, running elevates blood pressure to a substantial degree during exertion, and it is not necessarily recommended for persons with severe hypertension. If you are over forty, a physical examination and a stress test may be advisable before you begin to jog.

Third, not all city dwellers have immediate access to a park, and they may thus be forced to run on hard pavement in the midst of heavy traffic. Concrete is notoriously unfriendly to the hips, knees, and ankles, while the deep breaths runners take may contain volumes of car exhaust. If your city or town has a park or indoor cinder track, it makes good sense to confine your running to those locations.

All this said, it is also true that jogging is a time-honored aerobic exercise that produces one of the most exhilarating workouts possible.

Important: Before you start, acquire a good pair of running shoes. They will cushion your joints and make you feel pleasantly light on your feet as you run. Start modestly. Ten minutes a day is a good initial goal. It's best if you can run on earth or cinder track rather than on pavement. Increase your time to twenty or thirty minutes a day, three or four times a week. Running more than two or three miles a day is generally unnecessary and can even be counterproductive Remember, you are interested in reducing your blood pressure and getting in shape, not in marathon records (there is evidence to show that the super efforts made by long-distance runners increase stress hormones such as cortisol and epinephrine, temporarily depressing the immune system). A mile or two per jogging session is generally more than adequate for anyone over forty.

### Stair climbing

Stair climbing is another excellent aerobic exercise, especially if you live in a house or apartment with a staircase. Stair climbing produces wonderful cardiovascular benefits, though it can be hard on the knees and ankles. Stair-climbing gym machines tend to be a bit gentler in this regard. Start slowly, ten or fifteen minutes a day, and work up from there to a half hour or forty-five minutes a day, four times a week. But be warned: Using a stepping machine is notoriously boring. You may wish to ease the tedium by placing your machine in front of the TV.

### Rowing

Like cycling, rowing is predominately an upper-body exercise that strengthens the arms, shoulders, and chest. And as in cycling, the effects are well distributed, your cardiovascular health increases and many major organ systems are strengthened. If you have access to a boat and a navigable body of water, start with a half hour a day of rowing every three or four days, then build to forty-five minutes a day, then an hour. If you are exercising at home on a rowing machine, start with a thirty-minute workout three times a week (with the resistance level set to low), and build up to an hour a day four times a week (with increased resistance).

The following physical activities all offer excellent forms of exercise. They are not purely aerobic, however, since they do not involve continuous activity. While playing tennis, for example, you indulge in bursts of intense effort punctuated by moments of rest. All the activities listed below work the heart and lungs, increase endurance, and produce that sense of mental well-being that comes from intense physical exertion.

- basketball
- calisthenics
- golf
- handball
- ice skating
- martial arts
- racquetball
- roller skating
- squash
- tennis
- volleyball

## The Three Stages of Exercise

People often think of exercise as a kind of single explosive event that you do for a while and then stop. Actually, to derive maximum cardiovascular benefits, an aerobic workout is best approached in three stages:

1. warm-up period
2. main exercise
3. cooling-down period

### WARMING UP

The body, like most machines, is not built to go from a dead stop to full throttle without a gradual buildup. Indeed, launching into a sudden bout of intense exercise without working up to it can be hazardous to your health. Tendons can be pulled. Charley horses can cripple you for a week. And worse.

Always warm up.

As a rule of thumb, let your warm-up period equal approximately one-sixth of your entire exercise time.

This means that if you use a rowing machine for an hour a day, the first ten minutes should be spent loosening up. If you walk or jog a half hour a day, warm up with the proper calisthenics for a minimum of five minutes.

What constitutes a proper warmup?

Everybody has his or her pet methods, though there are certain basics to keep in mind. A good warm-up session should:

• discourage muscular and skeletal injuries by loosening and stretching the muscles, tendons, and ligaments;
• raise the heartbeat by slow degrees;
• gradually raise the breathing rate;

- gradually increase the body temperature;
- gradually speed up circulation.

Any good combination of stretches, bends, twists, and squats will accomplish these goals.

If, for example, your exercise of choice is calisthenics, warm up with a few gentle swings and twists, then gradually work your way up to the more demanding movements.

When jogging, start by stretching the hamstrings in your legs, touching your toes, and running in place for several minutes before setting off.

If you swim, begin your laps at half speed, breathing slowly and deeply. Then build up momentum as you go.

Above all, be gentle on your heart and circulatory system when you first begin. Since you are exercising to control your hypertension, you will want to be especially careful of overstimulating the cardiac system or raising your blood pressure too suddenly. Running in place, jumping jacks, treading water, half deep-knee bends—all are excellent for gradually raising the cardiovascular volume when you begin. Slow and steady wins the race here.

### THE MAIN EXERCISE

Once your body is warmed up, you will want to maximally condition your cardiovascular system and promote optimal health. The determining factors for accomplishing this are *exertion* during exercise, *duration of time* spent working out, and *frequency*—how often you exercise in a given week.

**Exertion**

Exertion is the degree of intensity reached during a workout; that is, how much effort and energy you expend while exercising. The key to determining this figure is to find your *target level heart rate*, the optimum speed at which your heart should beat during an exercise session. This speed should be fast enough to produce maximum conditioning but moderate enough to avoid causing harm.

Finding your target level heart rate is a two-stage operation:

*Stage one:* Determine your *maximum predicted heart rate*. For a person in good health, the quickest method of finding this figure is to subtract your current age from 220.

Example: if you are fifty years old, the calculation looks like this:

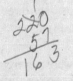

$$
\begin{array}{r}
220 \\
-50 \\
\hline
170 \text{ (your maximum}
\end{array}
$$
predicted heart rate)

If you are sixty-three years old, the calculation looks like this:

$$
\begin{array}{r}
220 \\
-63 \\
\hline
157 \text{ (your maximum}
\end{array}
$$
predicted heart rate)

*Stage two:* Now multiply your maximum predicted heart rate by .75.

In a fifty-year-old man, the calculation looks like this:

170 (maximum predicted heart rate)

× .75

127 (your target level heart rate during exercise if you are fifty years old)

And for a sixty-three-year-old:

157

× .75

117 (your target level heart rate during exercise if you are sixty-three years old)

Thus, if you a fifty-year-old man whose exercise of choice is fast walking, you will want to raise your pulse rate to approximately 127 to achieve optimum conditioning. Note that if you are over sixty years old and your fitness level is poor (or if you are taking up aerobic exercise for the first time), it's best to lower the .75 multiplier rate by ten points, to .65.

How do you measure your own pulse?

A simple and efficient method is to take your wrist pulse, count the number of beats that occur in a six-second period, and add a zero to this figure. In other words, if your pulse clocks in at eleven beats per six-second period during an exercise session, add a zero to the 11 for a pulse count of 110. If your pulse beats fourteen times in six seconds, add a zero to the 14 for a pulse rate of 140.

While there are more refined pulse-taking methods, this one is reliable enough for most people's purposes.

### Duration

Table 4 provides an approximate gauge of how long you should maintain a target level heart rate with a number of different exercises.

### Table 4: Duration of Exercise

| Exercise | Number of minutes to keep your heart at target level |
|---|---|
| Aerobic exercise | 15–20 |
| Calisthenics | 20–30 |
| Cycling | 15–30 |
| Dancing | 20–40 |
| Jogging | 15–30 |
| Rowing | 20–40 |
| Stair climbing | 15–30 |
| Swimming laps | 20–30 |
| Using treadmill | 15–30 |

Note: Check your pulse several times as you exercise to make sure you're in the right ballpark. If your pulse is lower than the target rate, increase your exercise intensity; if too high, slow down.

As your fitness level increases you may eventually wish to raise duration to the maximum levels. You be the judge here; just avoid pushing too hard. Moderate exercise consistently practiced is far better than pushing the envelope.

As a last consideration, you may wish to monitor your blood pressure before you exercise and then after. It's interesting to note how often pressure drops after a good workout and stays at that level for the rest of the day.

### Frequency

How often should you exercise?

Four times a week is ideal. If you work out less frequently, you take the chance of not giving your heart and circulatory system the conditioning they need. On the other hand, working out more often can be a strain unless you are physically fit. Some people simply alternate days, exercising one day, resting the next. This is an especially good method for people over forty.

#### COOLING DOWN

The final stage in the exercise process is really just warming up in reverse. After twenty or thirty minutes at maximum intensity, the body needs to decelerate by degrees. The heartbeat must be allowed to slow and the respiration rate return to normal. Cooling down is, in its own way, as important as warming up; wise exercisers try never to omit it.

As in warming up, each person has his or her favorite cooling-down techniques.

After a half-hour run, for example, some people walk the last five or ten minutes. Following a strenuous bout of aerobic dance, some people do gentle squats and toe touches, or they sit with their legs outstretched and gradually allow their head to drop to their knees. Whatever methods one chooses, the important thing to remember is that after a bout of intense exercise gradual slowing down is both more pleasant and more healthy than coming to a sudden stop.

"Within the past five years," writes Robert S. Eliot, M.D., in *From Stress to Strength*, "I personally have lost three apparently aerobically fit medical colleagues to sudden cardiac death because they did not progressively cool down."

According to Dr. Eliot, when an intense workout is stopped without a cool-down transition period, blood pools in the legs instead of returning to the heart, which is still pumping away at high-pitched exercise levels. Result? The amount of blood reaching the heart drops suddenly. This in turn can cause the heart to malfunction and, equally dangerous, cut off the blood supply to the brain (people who experience sudden light-headedness after abruptly ending an exercise are more than likely experiencing this effect).

"The cool-down period gives the arteries in your legs ample time to constrict steadily," writes Dr. Eliot, "shunting the blood from the lower extremities back to the heart. Meanwhile, as the heart rate slows, oxygen requirements diminish, and the entire system stabilizes. In essence, the cool-down should take about five minutes."

### Exercise: Some Important Things to Know

Crossing the exercise Rubicon and committing to a regular exercise program can be one of the most critical decisions you make in your life. Exercise works. It saves lives. At the same time, there are things you should know about exercising before making a commitment. The following suggestions are offered as food for thought:

*Avoid the most common exercise mistake—prolonged, infrequent sessions.* It's long been known to educators that we learn better if we study a topic for a moderate amount of time each day than if we try to stuff all the information into a single multihour cram session.

The same principle applies to exercise: a moderate workout practiced on a regular weekly schedule produces far better results than one long burst of intense exercise practiced once a week. Consistency and regular practice are far more important elements in the physical conditioning game than occasional heroic efforts.

*Moderate exercise can be as valuable as heavy.* High-intensity aerobic and resistance exercises such as swimming and bicycle riding are excellent tonics for cardiovascular health. At the same time, recent studies have demonstrated that light to moderate exercise also reduces cardiovascular risk. In the Harvard Alumni Study of 17,000 men, participants showed a reduced risk of coronary artery disease with as little as 500 calories per week expended in exercise. Consistency rather than intensity is the most important ingredient.

*Weight training can be helpful for blood pressure control if practiced with light hand weights and with a high number of repetitions.* As pointed out, weight lifting is mainly an isometric exercise, and at times can raise blood pressure to unacceptable levels. This is true, however, only when extremely heavy weights are used. New evidence suggests that weight-training programs using moderate-resistance weights with high numbers of repetitions—for example, 5- or 10-pound hand weights pressed ten or twenty times—are aerobically beneficial and physically safe.

In a recent clinical study of nine middle-aged patients who trained three times a week for twenty minutes every day using moderate-resistance weight exercises, none experienced compromised heart rate or abnormal blood pressure response.

Resistance training with light weights has also been shown to increase HDL cholesterol and to lower diastolic pressure. The key here is moderation with repetition.

*To maximize your workout, practice with a friend.* Studies have shown that exercisers who work out regularly with a friend stick to their training schedules more faithfully than those who go it alone. Working out with another person takes the tedium out of physical activity, makes the time go by more quickly, and allows both parties to help each other stick to their regimens.

*Exercise at the time that is best for you.* When is the best time of day to exercise? It all depends on your situation. Those who jog or work out in urban areas are advised to take their workouts in the early morning before rush hour traffic raises the air pollution level. Persons sensitive to heat should exercise in the morning before temperatures and humidity go too high. Time-of-day studies done at William Beaumont Hospital in Birmingham, Michigan, suggest that people who work out in the morning stick with their exercise program more faithfully than those who work out in the afternoon. Other people find that exercising in the afternoon helps them avoid "four o'clock slump." According to studies done at the Stanford Sleep Disorders Clinic in California, late afternoon is the best time of day to stretch the muscles, and just before bedtime the worst.

What does all this tell us? Basically, that there is no ideal hour of the day to exercise, and that people should pick their times according to their needs. Medical experts tend to agree that exercising in a consistent and determined way is far more important than working out at any special time of day.

*Turn ordinary daily activities into exercise opportunities.* Garden. Work in the yard. Take advantage of walking trails in a nearby park. Mow the lawn yourself instead of paying someone else to do the job. When you walk your dog, walk quickly and jog a small part of the way (your dog will love you for it). Walk to work instead of taking the car. If you take a bus or subway to work, get off a few stops early and walk the rest of the way. Play tennis, bowl, or golf instead of watching TV. Walk up stairs instead of taking the elevator. Take advantage of the long corridors at your local mall to do a bit of speed walking. If you work at a desk, stand up periodically, stretch, breathe deeply, and walk around the room.

In short, turn the ordinary activities of daily living

into exercise opportunities. The more you look for these opportunities, the more they will present themselves.

*Learn to recognize exercise danger signs.* According to studies done at the Miriam Hospital in Providence, Rhode Island, there is only one death per year from cardiac arrest for every 15,000 healthy joggers. Other studies record similarly low mortality rates. As far as exercise safety goes, the statistics are mightily on your side.

At the same time, as with paying attention to the safety briefings on an airplane before takeoff, it makes good common sense simply to be informed on the off chance that trouble comes along.

If, for example, you find yourself inappropriately out of breath or suddenly gasping for air while exercising, or if your pulse rises unnaturally high with severe palpitations and missed beats, stop at once and consult a physician. Sudden flushing, severe dizziness, nausea, and pain in the chest, jaw, or neck can all signal trouble.

If you jog or perform exercises that pound the joints, be sensitive to sudden or unusual pain in those parts. Don't strain, and never push beyond your limits. The once-popular adage "No pain, no gain" is largely out of favor today. In fact, pushing to the point of pain while exercising is counterproductive, and the pain may be your body's way of telling you you're overdoing.

It's sound policy to get a thorough physical checkup before beginning any exercise regimen.

### Step Three: Stress Reduction

**Keeping Your Blood Pressure Down by Keeping Your Stress Level under Control**

You don't need a complicated set of measuring devices to verify that stress raises your blood pressure. Just try this test. Next time you're feeling edgy or explosive, take your blood pressure and make a note of the figures.

Then wait until you're feeling more relaxed.

Check your pressure again. Chances are the numbers in the second reading are substantially lower than in the first.

Whether stress is a seminal cause of chronic hypertension or simply a temporary trigger is a question still being argued. What we do know is that even the small stressors of daily living can cause your blood pressure to rise by as much as 5 mm Hg or more—stressors such as hearing a loud noise, having a conversation with your boss, or cooking a meal. Conversely, relaxing at home or chatting with a friend produces an equivalent drop in pressure.

The physiological relationship between stress and blood pressure is not fully understood, though it appears to be associated with the fight-or-flight mechanism, that is, with the physiological reflex that responds to perceived dangers by either preparing for a struggle (fight) or running away (flight).

In premodern days these dangers might have included the attack of a wild animal or a fire in the forest. In our modern world they take the form of tax audits, lost reports at the office, tiffs with a spouse, and five-mile-long traffic jams.

Each time such a harassing episode occurs, our bodies respond by preparing for a bout of combat. The adrenal glands produce extra adrenaline and send it to the major organs in the body, speeding up circulation and causing the muscles to tense. Heart rate goes up accordingly, and breathing increases. The palms sweat. Appetite decreases. Blood cholesterol and blood sugar increase. And, of course, blood pressure rate rises.

The more anxiety-provoking the incident, the more feverishly the body works to prepare for it, and the higher the systolic and diastolic rates soar. The fact that real combat never comes, at least in the form of a physical struggle, is irrelevant to the fight-or-flight mechanism. In fact, the fight-or-flight mechanism *never* learns. No matter how many false alarms come its way over the years, over a lifetime, it continues to misread each incidental exasperation as a life-threatening event, and revs up the body's energies accordingly. Over the years, over a lifetime, this constant inappropriate stimulation wears us down.

Can controlling the levels of stress you experience each day at home and on the job help lower your blood pressure?

Probably. A majority of health care professionals now seem to think so, at any rate, and hypertensive patients across the country make successful use of a variety of stress-controlling methods. Exactly how much your blood pressure will decrease through the use of these stress-reduction techniques and how long it will stay at lower levels is difficult to say. Results depend on each individual's personality, lifestyle, and physical makeup. Chances are strong, however, that your blood pressure's health will profit from these routines, and that you will come to feel more relaxed and centered in the process.

The following nonpharmacological techniques are all powerful tools for quieting the mind, soothing the emotions, calming the body—and hence lowering blood pressure. You don't have to start using all these exercises at once. Run through the list, determine which methods are most compatible with your time demands and lifestyle, and give the ones you like a try.

### STRESS RELEASER ONE: RELAXATION THERAPY

While it is difficult to clinically evaluate exactly how many of our physical ills are worsened by body tension, it's widely acknowledged that formal relaxation techniques not only lower blood pressure but improve physiological functions such as sleep, digestion, and mental concentration. "The formula for perfect health is easy," an Asian tai chi teacher once told one of the authors. "It is relax, relax, relax."

The following two relaxation methods work best when practiced in the morning just after waking up and in the evening before going to bed. Find a quiet spot, sit or lie in a comfortable position, and put these routines to work. In the beginning you may wish to record your blood pressure before a session and then again after.

**Relaxation method one**

Lie on your back with arms at your sides and legs comfortably spread about twenty inches apart. Loosen any constricting clothing. Take several deep breaths and relax, eliminating all worrisome thoughts. Now start by concentrating on your forehead. Tense your scalp as tightly as possible and hold this tension for five to ten seconds. Then release. Feel the pleasant sensation of looseness in your head and neck. Blood circulation in this area is now stimulated, the muscles are slack, and an increment of bodily tension has been released.

Next, tense your forehead. Hold five to ten seconds. Release. Relax. Observe the pleasant sensations that follow.

Now the eyes. The nose (flare the nostrils and tighten the end of the nose). The mouth. The eyes. The back of the head. The chin. Enjoy the sense of relaxed warmth that follows each tightening.

Proceed in this manner down the length of your entire body. Tighten and release the neck. Likewise the shoulders, the chest, the upper arms, the lower arms, the wrists, hands, fingers, rib cage, stomach, abdomen, back (upper, middle, lower), hips, buttocks, groin, thighs, knees, calves, ankles, feet, and toes.

While untensing the different parts of your body, make certain that your mind is free of ordinary thoughts and worries. It's best to center your attention on the particular part of the body you're tightening and to keep mental activity at a minimum. Especially avoid negative thoughts. Disturbing mental images will produce tension and interfere with your attempts to relax.

It will take from five to ten minutes to move down the length of your body, depending on how much time you spend tightening each part. You can repeat the process as many times as you like. At the end of each session lie quietly for a few minutes, enjoying the benefits of physical and mental refreshment that follow. When you are ready to join the world again, take several deep breaths and slowly get up. Easy does it, now; you'll want to let the feelings of relaxation linger as long as possible.

### Relaxation method two

Sit in a comfortable chair with your back straight, hands on the your thighs, and feet resting firmly on the floor.

Take several deep breaths. Relax. Let go. Give in.

Starting at the top of your head, imagine that your body is filled with water, and that you are about to drain this water down through the length of your entire body and out of a hole on the bottom of each foot.

Begin by imagining that the water is starting to drain slowly downward from the top of your head. Watch as it drains down through your forehead and face, your neck and shoulders; down through your chest, abdomen, and hips; down through your thighs, calves, and ankles. Picture the water level dropping notch after notch. Feel the sensation of emptiness in the various parts of your body.

When the water line reaches your feet, imagine that the water is draining out through a hole in the middle of the sole of each foot. Let the water flow freely into the ground. Picture it gushing out like water from a hose.

Repeat the entire exercise.

After doing this exercise twice concentrate on the point in the center of your soles. Imagine that the water is continuing to run out. Keep your mind fixed on this flowing sensation. If you like, think of the water as tension. Picture it as a dark, murky fluid that is pouring out of you in streams, leaving you empty and relaxed.

Continue imagining this flow for five or ten minutes. At times you may feel a tingle in your feet or a sensation that something really is flowing through you. Go with this feeling. It means the exercise is doing its job. After a while you should enjoy a deep and increasing sense of serenity and release.

At the end of the session take several deep breaths and get up slowly. This exercise is effective anytime you're feeling anxious, frightened, or on edge. You can do it sitting on a chair at your desk, standing waiting for a bus, or when you're lying in bed at night.

### STRESS RELEASER TWO: DEEP BREATHING

Dr. Dean Ornish, a leading spokesman for the natural approach to cardiovascular health, remarks that "deep breathing is one of the simplest, yet most effective stress-management techniques there is."

At the Preventive Medicine Research Institute in Sausalito, California, Ornish and his associates have developed several highly effective stress and cardiovascular management programs that center on forms of breathing therapy, many of which are derived from the age-old principles of yoga.

You don't, of course, need to enroll in a health care institute to put deep breathing exercises to work. The following techniques can all be practiced at home or on the job whenever you're feeling tense. You'll be pleased to see how much deep breathing can calm you down, even in the most tense situations. Try the following:

• Whenever you have a quiet moment, sit in a chair with your back straight and practice five minutes of deep breathing. One simple exercise is as follows: Breathe in for a count of seven, hold your breath for a count of three, then exhale for a count of seven again. Do ten repetitions. Repeat this exercise when you wake up in the morning, when you start your day's work, at lunchtime, and in the afternoon. The good effects will influence your entire day.

• If you feel agitated or overwrought, stop what you're doing, relax, and take several deep breaths. Wait a few minutes, then take several more. This little trick alone can put you back on an emotional even keel. It can be practiced anytime you need it, even in moments of chaos and confusion. *Especially* in moments of chaos and confusion. There's an old saying: "Before you do anything rash, take ten deep breaths." Good advice.

• When practicing deep breathing, breathe first into your stomach, then into your midsection, and finally into your lower and upper chest. This breath is made in one single flowing motion: abdomen, midsection, lower chest, upper chest. Based on the principles of yoga, the "stomach breath" sees to it that your chest cavity is filled with air, that your lungs are properly exercised, and that oxygen intake is maximized.

• At various times during the day make a conscious effort to breathe more deeply and purposefully. Increasing the depth of your breathing even a little helps bring more oxygen into your system, and hence makes a noticeable difference in your overall stress level.

• Don't forget the importance of the out-breath. When performing deep breathing we tend to concentrate too heavily on inhaling, forgetting that a vigorous exhalation rids the lungs of stale air and removes toxins. To achieve maximum stress reduction, deep inhalation and deep exhalation are equally important.

• Program yourself to automatically take several deep breaths whenever a stressor goes off in your day's activities. For example, take several deep breaths when answering the phone, walking into a room full of strangers, meeting a significant new person, beginning a new task, or when the bottom falls out and others around you are going to pieces.

### STRESS RELEASER THREE: NATURAL REMEDIES

Although older civilizations have long used a variety of herbal potions to overcome tension and fatigue— and although European pharmacies have sold antistress herbal preparations for centuries—it's only in the past five or ten years that these remedies have found their way into the American medicine chest. Today, in fact, Americans embrace a wide range of herbal tranquilizers with perhaps a bit too much conviction, not always reading the labels on the bottles or bothering to question the claims made in the vitamin catalogs and health store ads. As with any health care item, buyers must be discerning in their choice of natural relaxants, acting out of knowledge rather than blind faith.

Which antistress herbs work best? Which potions really do calm us down and help keep blood pressure controlled? There are some definite standouts, all of which can be purchased at most health stores and pharmacies. These include:

**Valerian root**

A safe and powerful central nervous system depressant, valerian root has been used in China, Russia, and Europe for centuries as a specific against tension, depression, anxiety, hysteria, insomnia, and nervous conditions. Its effects are both sedative and tranquilizing.

In one Russian study, a tincture of valerian root was given to 23 men suffering from high blood pressure. The herb was shown to produce substantial tranquilizing effects in more than three quarters of participants. In another study, 128 insomniacs took an aqueous valerian root extract before bedtime. Next day a majority reported a deeper, better quality of sleep without the depressive side effects that can accompany chemical sedatives. Valerian root apparently does not cause secondary disorders. Even better, according to clinical studies it actually improves motor coordination and concentration, even as it reduces stress and tranquilizes the nervous system.

Do note, however, that for a small number of people valerian acts as a stimulant rather than a sedative. If you plan to try this herb, start off on a low dosage. If you feel calmer, as most people do, increase the dose. After two weeks, stop taking the valerian, wait several weeks, then begin again.

**St. John's Wort**

Another tried-and-true nervous disorder remedy, St. John's wort is a specific for depression, an ailment that is often accompanied by feelings of restlessness and anxiety.

This herb is among the most thoroughly tested natural medicines on the market today—one successful double-blind study of St. John's wort in Germany involved 3,250 subjects. Test results show that this herb has a powerful serotonin-boosting effect, and that for many people it works as well on bad moods as most prescription antidepressives. Yet unlike chemical antidepressives, St. John's wort is inexpensive and produces side effects in less than 1 percent of patients.

Even for individuals who are not clinically depressed, St. John's wort may be useful as a mood elevator and as a specific against the rigors of everyday tension. As a medicinal preparation it works best when taken in extract form standardized to 0.3 percent hypericin. The optimal safe and effective dosage, as determined in clinical tests, is 300 milligrams of the extract taken three times a day. Be sure to look for the phrase "0.3 percent hypericin" on the label.

**Kava-Kava**

An extract taken from the kava-kava plant, this highly effective herbal import has long been used in the South Pacific as the centerpiece for sacred communal ceremonies. Producing a tranquilizing effect, it is a specific against both stress and anxiety.

A 1996 study of twenty-nine patients reported in the journal *Phytomed* focused on patients diagnosed with a variety of anxiety disorders, including panic disorders and general tension. Given 100 mg of kava-kava extract three times a day for four weeks, subjects were evaluated according to three standard psychological profiles of anxiety. Most subjects were found to be measurably improved, and no side effects were reported. Kava-kava is becoming increasingly popular as a natural stress reliever in the West, and it can be purchased at most pharmacies and health product stores. The liquid extract is the most potent form, but it has a bitter taste. Capsules are easier on the taste buds but slightly less effective. It's your call.

### Chamomile

Not as powerful as valerian root or kava-kava, the lovely little chamomile bud still deserves an honored place among the antistress tools of the trade. Not only are its relaxing effects quickly felt, but it is useful for taming headaches, indigestion, and the symptoms of colds and flu. Studies indicate that in some cases the antispasmodic properties of chamomile, (when it is taken over a period of time) help prevent the development of ulcers, a condition directly linked to stress. You may wish to drink several cups of chamomile tea throughout the day, both at home and on the job, as a specific against the emotional ups and downs of daily living. The relaxing results are almost instantaneous. Be careful not to overdose on this substance, though; more than five or six cups a day can slow down motor reactions and produce feelings of sluggishness. Chamomile can be used as a tea, or it can be taken in capsule form. It is often a primary ingredient in antistress herbal mixtures.

**Other helpful stress releasers**

There are literally hundreds, perhaps thousands, of natural plant substances from around the world that help soothe the nervous system. Some of the more potent and readily available include:

fennel seed
hops
lavender flowers
lemon balm
linden flowers
passionflower
peppermint leaves
Siberian ginseng

### STRESS RELEASER FOUR: MEDITATION

Most of us have been bombarded with so many images of swami meditators on mountaintops that the real meaning of meditation has been lost. Meditation's roots lie in religion, it's true. But one does not have to be a Buddhist monk or even particularly spiritually minded to practice it. In its essence meditation is not prayer at all but a kind of mental calisthenic that takes whatever form and focus a meditator chooses to give it.

What does this calisthenic consist of?

In brief, the meditative act involves funneling one's awareness onto a single image, sound, or idea to the exclusion of all other thoughts and feelings. The object of concentration can be anything one chooses: a beautiful landscape, awareness of one's breath, even the mental repetition of a word like *peace* or *relax*. (One study determined that repeating to oneself a positive word that ends with an *m* or *n* sound—like *heaven* or *sun*—slows the heartbeat and causes blood pressure to drop.)

After meditators choose their object of focus, their goal is to keep this chosen image fixed in mind as steadily as possible without being diverted by habitual patterns of thought, daydreams, or discursive thinking.

Why would we want to make such an effort?

Because, as so many committed meditators have discovered, when the mind remains zoomed in on a single thought or image for an uninterrupted length of time a strange thing begins to take place. Not only does the clatter of the outside world recede, but a deeply refreshing sense of serenity and stillness fills the empty space, freeing meditators from daily cares and producing profound sensations of physical and mental unwinding.

If you have never meditated, you're in for a pleasant surprise. Here's a simple starter exercise to give you a taste of what it's all about.

**Meditation one**

Sit in a comfortable chair with your back straight. Take several deep breaths, close your eyes, relax, and slowly start to count: one, two, three, four. . . .

While counting, visualize each number as if it were written on a blackboard in front of you. Try not to allow other thoughts to enter your mind. Keep your concentration firmly fixed on the numbers.

Count slowly and purposefully from one to ten, then back again from ten to one.

If at any point in this process you lose your concentration and start thinking of other things, just pick up where you left off and continue. Practice this exercise for five to ten minutes every morning, and five to ten minutes every night. It seems overly simple at first, but when practiced regularly it can produce profound states of relaxation and well-being.

Once you feel comfortable with this exercise, try a more advanced meditation. For example:

**Meditation two**

Sit quietly with your back straight and eyes closed. Take several deep breaths, then center your awareness on your breathing.

Don't alter your chest or abdominal movements in any way. Simply breathe as you always do, keeping your mind fixed on the easy rhythms of the in-breath and out-breath. When your mind begins to wander, as it inevitably will, take note that you have lost concentration and return your attention to the breath.

Easier said than done? Absolutely. Did you lose your concentration again? And again? And again? Don't worry, everybody does. It's part of the process. Just remember, each time you make the effort to return your attention back to the breath your mind gets a little stronger and your body a little more relaxed. This exercise is especially useful at night before bed. It lets you unwind from a busy day, and helps you relax for a deeper sleep.

**Meditation three**

Sit comfortably with your back straight. Close your eyes and take several deep breaths.

In your mind's eye, picture a breathtakingly beautiful landscape. The landscape can be a place you've visited before, such as a garden, a mountain trail, a place by the sea. It can be your own original fantasyland. Or it can be a combination of both.

Imagine that you are walking through a large golden gateway, about to enter this wonderful domain. Smell the fragrant air. The sky is filled with birds. Listen to their song. Bask in the warmth of the sun and the beauty of the mountain peaks or open vistas surrounding you. Reach down and pick some flowers. Amble through a field of daisies till you come to a bubbling brook. Take off your shoes and wade in the water, stopping now and then to pick up a glittering gemstone, an emerald or a ruby. Climb a tree to a small, beautifully furnished house in the branches. Sit down on a large pillow. Take a refreshing drink from a sparkling carafe. Gaze out the window at the glorious landscape. Several musicians are sitting nearby holding strange, beautiful instruments. They start to play. Listen to the sublime music that surrounds you. Let go. Give in.

Continue building mind pictures in this vein, allowing your fantasy to take you where it will. Always keep your images bright, picturesque, and serene.

Each person will wish to create his or her own scenario. The important thing is that you let your imagination unfold on its own and carry you along, but at the same time, that you avoid losing your train of concentration. After a few minutes of wandering in your homemade pleasure garden you'll be reluctant to leave.

Ten- or fifteen-minute meditation sessions are long enough in the beginning. Some people set aside an area of their house or apartment for these sessions. That is fine. But remember, the significant thing about meditation is that you can practice it anytime you're feeling hassled and stressed. Just find a quiet place, close your eyes, take a few deep breaths, and plunge in. You'll be amazed how just ten or fifteen minutes of this ancient practice settles you down, quiets your nerves, sharpens your thinking—and in many cases lowers your blood pressure.

**STRESS RELEASER FIVE:**

**TWO ANCIENT METHODS FROM THE EAST**

We've already taken a close look at the relationship between exercise and hypertension, and it's clear that standard aerobic exercise is a powerful, multipronged tool for cardiovascular health. Here it should be added that besides conventional aerobic-style workouts, other, less rigorous exercise systems are also of value, specifically because of the emphasis they place on stress reduction. These exercises are the Eastern-based systems of yoga and tai chi.

Of the two methods, yoga is better known in the Western world and more widely practiced.

### Yoga

An age-old system of stretches, bends, breath control, and, at an advanced level, complex postures, yoga is designed to increase circulation, improve digestion, stimulate nerve energy, strengthen the joints and spine, and impart a tranquilizing effect. To quote the well-known yoga Vishnudevananda, "Just as water flows through an open tap, so energy flows into relaxed muscles."

Today yoga classes are given just about everywhere in the United States, in malls, colleges, hospitals, and health clubs. A session performed early in the morning generates relaxing effects that work their magic throughout the day, especially if the session is followed by a few minutes of meditation. Many businesses and corporations offer yoga as part of their recreational programs. In some states yoga therapy is accepted by medical insurance companies as a treatment for orthopedic problems.

Do, however, be sure that your teacher is a certified instructor from a recognized training center, and that all exercises are compatible with the safety standards set by orthopedists and physical therapists. As with any exercise system, a period of warm-up and one of cooldown is essential for every session. Good teachers include these in the workout.

Once you learn the fundamentals, yoga can also be practiced at home on your own. Do be careful, however, of the pretzel-type positions you see illustrated in books. These can trigger serious back or joint damage and are for advanced exercisers only. If you are a beginner, stick to the elementary exercises, work with a certified teacher, and proceed at a moderate pace.

## Tai chi

A less popular but equally effective stress buster is the Chinese system of tai chi chuan, usually called simply tai chi. Perhaps you've seen men and women practicing this slow, graceful series of movements in a nearby park, or witnessed scenes on TV of people in Beijing performing their morning tai chi workout.

Though it seems strange that such slow, languid maneuvers can produce vitality and relaxation, this ancient set of movements has been developed by Chinese masters through the centuries to stimulate every organ and muscle in the body, and to circulate the subtle inner energies that the Chinese refer to as *chi*. The very act of performing such slow, purposeful movements causes the muscles and joints to work overtime. Try, for example, quickly raising your right arm above your head. Now try raising it very slowly. Which movement takes the greater effort? Which movement feels more relaxing when you're through?

Most people vote for the second. As one practitioner of tai chi remarked after an intense forty-five minute session, "I feel both like I just ran the marathon and just took a nap."

Although some people learn tai chi from illustrated books, if you plan to investigate this wonderfully relaxing exercise it's recommended that you study with a certified teacher. Tai chi schools exist in many areas of the country today, even rural areas, and the monthly cost is usually a good deal less than joining a gym. Try it and see.

Any words we hear repeated over and over we eventually start to believe.

This is the basis of brainwashing, of course, but the same principle can be applied in positive therapeutic ways, namely through the process of autohypnosis, or as it is sometimes referred to, self-suggestion.

Autohypnosis employs deep, self-induced relaxation to produce a light state of trance. Once this state is achieved, subjects give themselves a series of helpful suggestions—in this case, suggestions to unwind and relax. After the person comes out of the trance, these suggestions go to work on a subliminal level, influencing his or her daily behavior in subtle but real ways.

How safe is autohypnosis?

Despite sensational images of mad hypnotists controlling zombified victims, self-suggestion has been prescribed safely by mental health professionals for years. The strategy behind it is simple. Once relaxed, the theory goes, the deeper parts of the mind are more readily accessible than in the ordinary waking state, and the brain becomes more receptive to whatever advice we give it. In other words, by suspending the mental processes, and by putting body and mind in a quiescent state it's possible to bypass the ordinary defense mechanisms of the ego and talk directly to the unconscious.

Let's walk through a sample exercise in autosuggestion step by step, concentrating on stress control.

*Step one:* Sit or lie in a comfortable position with

your eyes open. Repeat to yourself your own version of the following message:

My eyelids are getting heavy. Very heavy. Heavier and heavier. They are beginning to close. Each lid seems to have a weight on it. They're closing, slowly and steadily. Closing. My eyelids are getting heavy. Very heavy. Heavier and heavier. So heavy they're starting to close. I'm getting more and more relaxed and sleepy as my eyes start to close. My eyes are closing now, more and more. I can feel them flickering. This is a sign that they are beginning to close. Heavier and heavier. Lower and lower. My eyes are starting to close now, more and more. Heavier and heavier . . .

*Step two:* Continue in this vein until your eyelids flutter shut. For most people this process takes no more than three or four minutes (you may be surprised to see how quickly you respond). When your lids drop, this is the first sign that the self-hypnosis is working.

Continue putting yourself into a state of deep relaxation with your own version of the following message:

My body is feeling very relaxed. Extremely relaxed. I am relaxing deeply. My face is relaxed. My neck and chest are relaxed. My arms. My stomach and legs. All very, very relaxed. Very heavy and relaxed. My arms and legs feel very heavy. It's as if they're sinking into the bed [chair, sofa]. Very heavy. Now that my eyes are closed I am sinking more and more into a deep, quiet state where nothing in the world can hurt or bother me. I am totally at peace. I am sinking deeper and deeper, totally relaxed and absorbed. Outside noises and disturbances do not affect me in the slightest way now. I feel so pleasantly drowsy, so comfortable, so happy. I am relaxing more and more, sinking more and more with every breath I take. My whole body has become very heavy. The outside world is disappearing. Every part of my body is relaxed now. My arms . . . my hands . . . my neck . . . the back of my head . . . my eyebrows . . . my elbows . . . my chest . . . my stomach . . . my knees . . . my feet . . . everything. I feel as if I'm sinking into the bed [chair, sofa], getting heavier and heavier. So relaxed now. I could move if I wanted to. But I don't want to. Because I am too comfortable and relaxed. The only thing I want to do now is relax. More and more. My arms are so pleasantly heavy. My legs. My head. All so comfortably heavy and still. Nothing bothers me now. My problems are all far, far away. Nothing can bother me now, nothing can touch me, nothing can disturb me or worry me, nothing can disturb me. The deeper I go, the more pleasant and relaxed I feel. . . .

This series of suggestions takes about five or ten minutes to achieve maximum effectiveness. Don't look for unconsciousness or rigidity as a sign that the suggestions are taking effect. On the contrary, you will experience a strange sense of alertness, but it will be coupled with a pleasant feeling of separation from the outer world.

You are now in a state of light autohypnosis and ready to take the next step.

*Step three:* Imagine that you are standing at the top of a long flight of stairs.

Peer down these stairs. See how they lead down, down, down, into a deep but hospitable darkness. Tell yourself that you are now going to walk down these stairs, and that each step you take will bring you deeper and deeper into self-hypnosis, deeper into relaxation.

Start down the stairs. Let each step sink you a little deeper. Proceed one step at a time until you reach the tenth step. Stop here at a landing.

Pause at the landing in a state of relaxation. Look back up the stairs and see how far you've come. Feel how deep your concentration is becoming.

Now walk down another ten steps and pause again at the next landing. Then walk down a third flight, letting yourself sink deeper and deeper as you go.

At the bottom landing tell yourself that you have arrived. Your mind is now open and receptive enough to start the process of self-suggestion.

*Step four:* All advice you give yourself in a state of autohypnosis should be simple, gentle, polite, totally positive, and never overly directive. Suggest, don't command. Something like:

I will be feeling more and more relaxed now in my daily life. Better and better. I like feeling relaxed during the day. It allows me to get my work done more effectively, and to keep my blood pressure under control. I like avoiding stress whenever I can. When I come out of this exercise, I will feel wonderful and will remain this way for the rest of the day. Very relaxed and at ease. There will not be any need for my blood pressure to rise. I will be completely relaxed and in control wherever I go and whatever I do. It's better to be relaxed than stressed. . . .

Recite a version of this message to yourself once or twice. No need to repeat it over and over again as you did when putting yourself into autohypnosis. Your unconscious is more open than usual now and will quickly get the gist. A few well-phrased suggestions will do the trick.

To give these suggestions increased clout, you may wish to support them with complementary mental images. For example, as you give yourself suggestions to relax at work, imagine yourself talking easily to others on the job, looking completely relaxed and in command. See yourself walking down a sunny street feeling wonderful. The sky is blue. Flowers are blooming. You are utterly unworried and serene. This combination of verbal guidance and visual imagery forms a synergetic effect that is more persuasive and powerful than the sum of its parts.

Continue giving yourself suggestions for two or three minutes, then end the session in the following way.

*Step five:* Imagine that you are standing at the bottom landing of the dark staircase, looking up. Imagine that you are about to climb the stairs, and that with each step you bring yourself closer to normal consciousness.

Start up the thirty steps slowly, rising step by step. When you reach the top tell yourself that you are now out of autohypnosis, perfectly normal, and ready to go about your business in a relaxed and positive way.

Practice this exercise daily, preferably at the same time each day. You may wish to prerecord your monologue, complete with suggestions, on a cassette tape, and play the tape back during each session. This method allows you to remain passive and receptive during the session without the need to speak.

Finally, it should be mentioned that this program is useful for other common disorders besides stress, such as simple insomnia, fatigue, worry, and even physical ailments like sore neck or painful back.

### STRESS RELEASER SEVEN: ASSORTED TRICKS AND TECHNIQUES FOR BETTER RELAXATION

### Don't work so hard

Easier said than done perhaps, but there are small steps you can take to combat workaholism. For example, make it a policy not to work on the weekends. Take five or ten minutes every day at your workplace to meditate and clear your head. Leave the job ten minutes earlier than usual several days a week. Don't take on extra projects if you can help it. Stop thinking so much about your job after quitting time. Don't bring home more office work than you have to. Take a day off now and then. If you have a sedentary job, make a conscious effort three or four times each day to stretch, breathe deeply, and relax at your desk. Slow things down—stress is never relieved by going faster, only by going slower.

### Cultivate a hobby

Sounds trite, but clinical studies show that people who practice a hobby tend to be more relaxed and feel more fulfilled. What kind of hobby? Anything that captures your fancy: sewing, carpentry, cooking, computers, hiking, gardening, stamp collecting, learning a new language. The idea is to become involved in a pastime that takes you out of yourself, gives you a sense of accomplishment, and lets you unwind.

Do, however, be careful not to approach your hobby as a competitive sport. Hobbies help the blood pressure *only* when done for the love of the hobby itself. If you learn to play the piano, do so for the sake of musical enjoyment, not to become the best pianist on your block. If you start a book collection, don't worry about building the best library in town, just enjoy the books for their own sake. Do what you love; the rewards will follow.

### Calm down with self-massage

Whenever you're tense lay on the hands—your own in this case. The following techniques are all effective measures for self-relaxation.

• Massage your hands, both the palms and the backs, and pull each finger for ten seconds.

• Rub your scalp and the back of your head and neck.

• Massage the area behind your knees.

• Slowly rotate your head clockwise two turns and then counterclockwise two turns, allowing your head to relax and droop by its own weight as you move it. The idea is that the weight of your head is both leading the movement and resisting it. Several minutes of this exercise will relax you deeply.

• Vigorously massage the soles of your feet, paying special attention to the sore spots and tender joints. Also massage the tops of your feet, and your ankles. If you enjoy the sensations this massage produces you may wish to purchase a book or pamphlet on foot reflexology to learn more. Books on the subject are available from most health product vendors.

• Rub your shoulders and neck. Use the left hand to rub the right shoulder and the right hand to rub the left shoulder. Continue the massage up the back of your neck with both hands.

• Make a fist and massage the mound between the thumb and first finger. Repeat for the other hand. This mound is a major acupressure point, and for many people rubbing it induces a relaxation response.

**Try water therapy**

Whenever you're feeling especially tense, soak your feet in several inches of hot water for twenty minutes. Cold baths (or showers) are also a remedy for nerves, and can work wonders when all else fails. And don't minimize the effects of a good swim at a local health club or YMCA for calming down and loosening up. Some people unwind at night with hot baths, also a good idea. But be warned: Hot baths taken immediately before getting into bed raise the body temperature and make it difficult to fall asleep. If you enjoy hot baths at night, climb in and out of the tub at least two hours before bedtime.

### Get up, get out

When things go wrong and you feel like you're going to fly out of your skin, don't just sit there. Get up, go out, break the mold, change the scene. Altering your environment when the roof is falling in is a proven antistressor. Instead of stewing in a chair for hours over a problem, try exercising. Or go shopping. Catch up on your gardening. Have a game of tennis. Take in a movie. Play with your children. Visit a friend. Take a walk—and a vigorous one at that. (Studies show that walkers who swing their arms and take long strides feel more relaxed than those who merely shuffle along.) The bottom line is that when things go wrong it's better to *do something*, anything at all, than to remain a passive victim.

### Don't keep it all bottled up

We now know that keeping our emotions stifled for too long is bad for the health. Repressed feelings raise blood pressure, trigger headaches, encourage ulcers, and bring on stomach distress, among other things. Better to let it out and let it go. You don't have to walk around yelling at everyone in sight, of course. Be discreet. In certain confrontational situations, however, it's sometimes better to take the risk and say what you think in a direct and uncompromising way—this, instead of beating around the bush and swallowing your anger.

Learn to initiate frank dialogues with people who cause you stress. Talk it out. Be courteous but direct. When you're feeling bad, say so, both to yourself and to others. The same holds true when you're by yourself. If you feel like crying, moaning, punching the pillow, complaining out loud, even yelling in the shower, go ahead and let fly. It's okay to hurt. There's nothing improper or "crazy" about these activities, and in many cases the sense of release they generate helps clear your psychological air.

# PART III

## Nutritional and Dietary Aids for Controlling Hypertension

# 4

## The Salt Connection

### Salt and Your Blood Pressure

We were all taught in school that salt is an essential nutrient, and that our bodies cannot do without it. You may remember being told how in ages past nations went to war over salt, or how in countries like Tibet where salt is scarce, it is sometimes used as a form of money. In Greece, a hardworking slave was said to be "worth his weight in salt." In Rome, a portion of a legionnaire's monthly wage was paid in bricks of salt (the word *salary* is derived from the Latin word *salarium*, or "salt money").

What makes salt, or sodium, as it is often called, so important to human functioning?

For one thing, it regulates the amounts of water that our bodies retain, governing the passage of fluid into and out of the cells, and helping the cell membranes remain elastic. Salt is needed by the digestive system for the metabolism of carbohydrates and proteins, and by the nervous system to aid in the transmission of nerve impulses. It is a basic ingredient in maintaining the electrolyte balance of the body and it plays an essential role in muscle contraction. Without an adequate supply of sodium in the body, muscle weakness, nausea, even heart problems can occur.

Clearly it's an important nutrient. But how much do we really need each day for it to do its job?

Not very much.

Understand that while the words *salt* and *sodium* are often used interchangeably, there is a difference between the two. In the language of chemistry, the table salt we're familiar with is termed *sodium chloride*. Only 40 percent of this crystal compound is sodium; the remaining 60 percent is chloride. This means that if you eat 10 grams of table salt a day you are actually receiving 4 grams of sodium. It is the sodium in the salt compound that precipitates factors that lead to high blood pressure.

Now according to standard health research, no more than a gram of sodium a day is necessary for the body to function properly. That's less than a teaspoonful of table salt daily. Ingesting more than this produces no known benefits. Yet the average American eats from *8 to 12 grams of table salt every day*, and often more. A single dinner of, say, tomato soup, creamed chipped beef, canned corn, mashed potatoes, salad with dressing, pickles on the side, and apple pie with cheddar cheese can add up to 7 or 8 grams. This is not to mention the breakfast, lunch, and snacks that precede it.

What effect does all this extra sodium have on our bodies?

In most cases, salt residues are filtered out by the

kidneys, voided through the urine, and that's that. No harm done.

But in people who are "salt-sensitive," a category believed to include from 30 to 50 percent of hypertensives (and populated heavily by people who are black, overweight, diabetic, and elderly), the kidneys do not eliminate salt as efficiently as they should. This deficiency causes extra water to build up in the body. The volume of blood increases in the blood vessels, and this places an added burden on the circulatory system. The heart, in turn, pumps more intensely and the blood vessels constrict.

Final result: elevated blood pressure.

Just how high a person's blood pressure can be forced up from excessive salt intake is a matter of individual sensitivity. Indeed, salt's precise effect on blood pressure remains something of an enigma to researchers, and no instrument has yet been invented to measure its full influence. The many studies done on the subject have produced mixed findings.

We know, for example, that in countries like New Guinea and in the jungle basins of Brazil, where salt is almost never used, high blood pressure simply does not exist. And that in the eastern areas of Canada, especially in Newfoundland, where a diet of salty fish is made all the more sodium-laden by traditional cooking practices, the mean average blood pressure of the local population is inordinately high.

On the other hand, farmers in northern Thailand ingest heroic quantities of salt on a daily basis, yet their blood pressures remain stable. And in the famous Framingham Heart Study, one of the most thorough and well-designed studies of American cardiovascular health patterns ever carried out, statistics show that hypertensive persons do not necessarily consume more salt than those with normal readings. There are many similarly contradictory findings.

What, then, is the consensus?

The consensus is that despite ambiguous evidence, a portion of the population is definitely more salt-sensitive than others, and that Americans tend to fall into the salt-sensitive category with something of a vengeance.

Few doctors today would deny that salt reduction is a significant mode of treatment for hypertensive patients, or that for many people this method is the best first line of defense. Certainly anyone who suffers from hypertension is well advised to try a low-sodium diet for at least three months and to measure the results. For some hypertensives, sodium reduction alone can normalize blood pressure.

It could then be asked why, if cutting back on salt is so effective, everyone with high blood pressure does not avail himself or herself of this simple strategy.

The usual answer is that salt is an addictive substance, and that going off it cold turkey is as difficult as, say, giving up smoking.

But this is nonsense. While salt is a mildly addictive substance, perhaps, cutting back is not only doable for most people but surprisingly easy, especially if it is carried out in stages. Even inveterate salt users discover that the habit can be tamed in a few weeks and broken in a few months. After a half year of low sodium, many ex-addicts find that they now prefer the taste of unsalted meats and vegetables, and that added salt gives their food a disagreeably strong and acrid taste.

Monitoring salt intake, what's more, delivers several secondary gains for hypertensives, specifically in the area of weight control. Fat cells, we know, tend to retain salt, and salt holds water. When salt intake is restricted, water retention is correspondingly reduced, causing the body to shed excess weight, and the fat cells to become smaller and fewer. There is also evidence to show that as we grow older our kidneys become less efficient at filtering salt, and that tolerance for this substance decreases as the years pass—another reason why people over fifty should watch their daily intake.

Excessive salt use, in short, is an acquired habit that brings few physical benefits, and that for salt-sensitive people can cause measurable harm. Breaking the habit is relatively easy, defies no known law of nature, and is strongly recommended for anyone who seriously wishes to control his or her hypertension.

## What They Don't Tell You about Hidden Salt in Your Food

The first requirement for maintaining a restricted salt diet is learning the salt content of everyday foods. What you find out here may surprise you.

For example, which of the following items do you think contains the largest amount of salt?

- a slice of commercial lemon meringue pie
- an ounce of salted peanuts
- a serving of fast-food french fries
- a pound of broiled sirloin steak

The answer: a slice of lemon meringue pie.

Why?

Because when a commercial pastry is produced its manufacturers know that several weeks and sometimes several months will elapse between the time the pie leaves the bakery and the time it's purchased at the store. To keep their product from spoiling, they are obliged to add a host of preservatives, many of them containing salt. Commercial bakers also know that certain additives catalyze the yeast during the baking process and enhance the color and savoriness of the crust. These too go into the vat.

The result: a host of salt-laden chemicals in your favorite cakes and pies.

How much sodium do our bodies actually reap from the preservatives found in commercial foods?

Hypertension specialist Thomas G. Pickering, M.D., has studied this subject in depth. In his book *Good News about High Blood Pressure*, he tells us that sodium finds its way into our food supply in five ways:

- through the local water supply
- through the salt found naturally in the raw ingredients we eat every day—vegetables, fruits, grains, dairy products, oils, and meats
- through salt added at the table

- through salt added to food during the cooking process
- through salt found in commercial additives, flavorings, and preservatives

Of these five sources, according to Dr. Pickering, water adds less than 1 percent of salt to our diet, raw ingredients account for 12 percent, salt added at the table provides 6 percent, cooking contributes 5 percent.

This means, Dr. Pickering tells us, that 77 percent— yes, 77 percent—of the sodium we take into our bodies is delivered by commercial additives, flavorings, and preservatives. This is a broad estimate, and just one doctor's estimate, mind you. But it is certainly worth thinking about.

Which specific preservatives are responsible for importing sodium into our diets?

All substances with the word *sodium* in them, and a few without. A short list of the usual suspects includes:

- *Sodium derivatives*. A partial sampling of sodium-based food additives includes sodium cyclamate (soft drinks), sodium sulfite (preserved fruits), sodium citrate (drinks, desserts), sodium propionate (antimold in cheese), sodium nitrate (meats), sodium nitrite (meats), sodium saccharin (sweetener), sodium caseinate (ice cream), sodium hydroxide (fruit and vegetable skin softener), and sodium benzoate (condiments, dressings).
- *MSG (monosodium glutamate)*. The controversial flavoring used to tenderize meat and enhance the flavor of food (especially at oriental restaurants and

in frozen dinners) is loaded with salt and salt-derived chemicals.

- *Dry skim milk.* Dry skim milk, used in home recipes and touted as a cardiovascular aid because of its low fat content, is heavy in salt.
- *Baking powder.* This widely used and seemingly innocuous kitchen favorite is loaded with sodium.
- *Brine.* Used to pickle, marinate, purify, and preserve foods like sauerkraut, pickles, olives, feta cheese, tomatoes, peppers, and corned beef, brine is as salty as seawater.

There are many others.

What do we do, then, to cut back on salt? How can we avoid the relentless bombardment of this substance, both in the additives that arrive on our plate hidden in commercial foods and in the supplies that reach us via tap water, raw ingredients, salt added at the table, and salt used during the cooking process?

The following section will guide you through these narrow straits, providing practical techniques to get your low-salt diet up and running, and to familiarize you with the vocabulary of low-salt living.

## Secrets of Maintaining a Low-Salt Diet

### 1. Avoiding salt in the water supply

The national average of 1 percent of salt in the water supply is so small that you usually don't need to worry about tap water interfering with your low-sodium diet.

Yet 1 percent is just an average. In some parts of the country, especially in the Southern and Southwestern states, groundwater contains unusually high amounts of sodium and is a significant source of ingested salt. If you live in one of these areas, consider having your water tested by a municipal water company or by an independent lab. Samples should show no more than 45 to 50 parts salt per million. If the local salt content turns out to be higher, switch to bottled water. Or consider purchasing a good under-the-sink water filter.

Beware too of commercial water softeners. The chemicals used in water-softening appliances generate a good deal of salt, and residues go directly into the water. If you are contemplating installing a water softener, ask the manufacturer for specs on the amount of sodium its product generates. If the count seems too high it may be best to stick with the hard water you presently use. Hard water is, as a number of clinical studies bear out, a good deal better for your cardiovascular health than soft.

## 2. Avoiding salt in the foods you eat every day

The first step in taming the salt habit is to familiarize yourself with the sodium content of your favorite foods, both raw and processed.

This doesn't mean you must measure in milligrams the precise sodium count of everything you eat. Most people find this method tedious and usually abandon it after a couple of days. Like calorie counting, all you really need are ballpark estimates. The question to ask first is whether a food has a:

- very high salt content—500 mg and over
- high salt content—300 to 500 mg
- medium salt content—between 150 and 300 mg
- low salt content—between 50 and 150 mg
- very low salt content—below 50 mg

Once familiar with these ranges you can plan your meals accordingly. Table 5 provides a broad sampling of the salt content in a number of common raw and processed foods.

### Table 5: Salt Content of Common Foods

| Food | Amount | Sodium (milligrams) |
|------|--------|---------------------|
| **Beverages** | | |
| Beer | 1 cup | 17 |
| Chicken soup, canned | 1 cup | 887 |
| Clam chowder, canned | 1 cup | 1,000 |
| Club soda | 1 cup | 59 |
| Coffee | 1 cup | 2 |
| Diet cola | 1 cup | 26 |
| Lentil soup, commercial | 1 cup | 859 |
| Tea | 1 cup | 1 |
| Tomato juice, commercial | 1 cup | 744 |
| Tomato soup, canned | 1 cup | 1,050 |

| Food | Amount | Sodium (milligrams) |
| --- | --- | --- |
| **Breads, cereals, grains, pasta** | | |
| Bagel | 1 medium | 310 |
| Bread, French | 1 slice | 120 |
| Bread, pumpernickel | 1 slice | 200 |
| Bread, rye | 1 slice | 129 |
| Bread, white | 1 slice | 118 |
| Bread, whole wheat | 1 slice | 125 |
| Bread stuffing mix | 1 cup | 1,008 |
| Bulgur, cooked | 1 cup | 1,498 |
| Cereal, Corn Chex | 1 ounce | 330 |
| Cereal, cornflakes | 1 ounce | 320 |
| Cereal, Cream of Wheat, instant | 1 cup | 10 |
| Cereal, granola | 1 cup | 300 |
| Cereal, oatmeal, instant | 1 cup | 250 |
| Cereal, oatmeal, regular | 1 cup | 5 |
| Macaroni and cheese | 1 cup | 2,000 |
| Muffin | 1 medium | 220 |
| Pizza, with cheese and sausage | 1 slice | 730 |
| Rice, brown | 1 cup | 423 |
| Rice, white | 1 cup | 512 |
| Roll, dinner | 1 medium | 190 |
| Roll, hot dog | 1 | 202 |
| Spaghetti, with meat sauce | 1 cup | 1,025 |
| Waffle | 1 average | 360 |
| **Dairy products** | | |
| Butter | 1 tablespoon | 116 |
| Buttermilk | 8 ounces | 257 |

| Food | Amount | Sodium (milligrams) |
|---|---|---|
| Cheese, American | 1 slice | 320 |
| Cheese, blue | 1 ounce | 396 |
| Cheese, Brie | 1 ounce | 178 |
| Cheese, cheddar | 1 slice | 200 |
| Cheese, cottage, low-fat | 1 cup | 430 |
| Cheese, cottage, whole-milk | 1 cup | 515 |
| Cheese, cream | 1 ounce | 85 |
| Cheese, mozzarella | 1 ounce | 220 |
| Cheese, Muenster | 1 ounce | 174 |
| Cheese, Swiss | 1 ounce | 74 |
| Cheese fondue | 1 pound | 2,455 |
| Cream | 1 cup | 110 |
| Cream, half-and-half | 1 tablespoon | 6 |
| Cream, sour | 1 tablespoon | 6 |
| Cream, whipped | 1 tablespoon | 3 |
| Egg, boiled | 1 medium | 60 |
| Egg, fried | 1 medium | 169 |
| Egg, yolk only | 1 medium | 14 |
| Ice cream | 1 cup | 100 |
| Milk, goat's | 1 cup | 80 |
| Milk, 1% | 8 ounces | 123 |
| Milk, skim, dry | 1 cup | 670 |
| Milk, 2% | 8 ounces | 122 |
| Milk, whole | 1 cup | 130 |
| Milk, whole, dry | 1 cup | 420 |
| Yogurt | 1 container | 120 |
| **Fish and seafood** | | |
| Bass | 1 pound | 240 |
| Bluefish | 1 pound | 470 |
| Clams, in shell | 1 pound | 510 |

| Food | Amount | Sodium (milligrams) |
|------|--------|---------------------|
| Cod, broiled | 1 pound | 506 |
| Crab | 1 pound | 3,850 |
| Flounder, baked | 1 pound | 1,090 |
| Haddock | 1 pound | 1,390 |
| Halibut | 1 pound | 255 |
| Lobster | 1 pound | 430 |
| Mackerel | 1 pound | 135 |
| Oysters, in shell | 1 pound | 369 |
| Salmon, fresh | 1 pound | 520 |
| Salmon, smoked | 1 pound | 2,354 |
| Sardines, drained | 3 ounces | 552 |
| Shrimp, canned | 1 pound | 4,999 |
| Shrimp, raw | 1 pound | 421 |
| Snapper | 1 pound | 161 |
| Trout | 3 ounces | 67 |
| Tuna, canned, in oil | 3 ounces | 303 |
| **Fruits** | | |
| Apple | 1 medium | 1 |
| Apricot | 1 medium | 2 |
| Avocado | 1 medium | 24 |
| Banana | 1 medium | 1.5 |
| Berries (blackberries, blueberries, cranberries, raspberries, strawberries) | 1 cup | 0 |
| Cantaloupe | ¼ cup | 12 |
| Cherries | 1 cup | 1 |
| Dates | 10 | 1 |
| Fig | 1 | 2 |
| Grapefruit | 1 medium | 2 |

| Food | Amount | Sodium (milligrams) |
|---|---|---|
| Grapes | 1 cup | 5 |
| Honeydew | 1 cup | 30 |
| Kiwi | 1 medium | 5 |
| Mango | 1 cup | 1 |
| Nectarine | 1 cup | 0 |
| Orange | 1 medium | 2 |
| Peach | 1 medium | 5 |
| Pear | 1 medium | 2 |
| Pineapple | 1 slice | 1 |
| Raisins | 1 cup | 17 |
| Tangerine | 1 cup | 0 |
| Watermelon | 1 large | 2 |
| **Meats and poultry** | | |
| Beef, dried chipped | 1 ounce | 944 |
| Beef, corned | ½ cup | 7,882 |
| Beef, corned beef hash | 1 cup | 1,520 |
| Beef, hamburger (from fast-food outlet) | 1 medium | 750 |
| Beef, hamburger (made with low-fat beef) | 1 medium | 100 |
| Beef, hot dog | 1 | 639 |
| Beef, lean | 1 pound | 215 |
| Beef, meat loaf TV dinner | 1 dinner | 1,304 |
| Beef, roast beef sandwich | 1 | 588 |
| Beef, sirloin steak | 1 pound | 230 |
| Beef, Swiss steak TV dinner | 1 dinner | 682 |

| Food | Amount | Sodium (milligrams) |
|---|---|---|
| Chicken, boiled | ½ breast | 47 |
| Chicken, fried | 1 pound | 300 |
| Chicken, roast | ½ breast | 69 |
| Chicken, TV dinner | 1 dinner | 1,153 |
| Chicken chow mein | 1 cup | 718 |
| Chicken pot pie (individual portion) | 1 | 594 |
| Duck, roast | ½ duck | 227 |
| Lamb, chops | 1 pound | 205 |
| Lamb, roast leg of | 1 pound | 199 |
| Lunch meat, bologna | 1 slice | 310 |
| Lunch meat, olive loaf | 1 slice | 312 |
| Lunch meat, pastrami | 3 ounces | 810 |
| Pork, bacon | 1 pound | 4,625 |
| Pork, chops | 1 pound | 300 |
| Pork, ham, cured | 1 pound | 3,252 |
| Sausage, pepperoni | 1 slice | 122 |
| Sausage, salami (pork-and-beef mix) | 1 slice | 217 |
| Turkey, roast | 1 pound | 450 |
| Turkey, TV dinner | 1 dinner | 1,228 |
| Turkey pot pie (individual portion) | 1 | 620 |
| Veal | 1 pound | 245 |
| Veal parmigiana | 7.5 ounces | 1,825 |
| **Oils** | | |
| Canola | 1 tablespoon | 0 |
| Corn | 1 tablespoon | 0 |
| Hydrogenated cooking fat | ½ cup | 1,115 |

| Food | Amount | Sodium (milligrams) |
|------|--------|---------------------|
| Lard | 1 tablespoon | 139 |
| Margarine | 1 tablespoon | 153 |
| Olive | 1 tablespoon | 0 |
| Peanut | 1 tablespoon | 0 |
| Safflower | 1 tablespoon | 0 |
| Sesame | 1 tablespoon | 0 |
| **Snacks, condiments, dressings** | | |
| Chili sauce | 1 tablespoon | 223 |
| Dressing, blue cheese | 1 tablespoon | 150 |
| Dressing, French | 1 tablespoon | 206 |
| Dressing, Italian | 1 tablespoon | 315 |
| Dressing, Russian | 1 tablespoon | 130 |
| Ketchup | 1 tablespoon | 180 |
| Mayonnaise | 1 tablespoon | 80 |
| Mustard, yellow | 1 tablespoon | 150 |
| Peanut butter | 1 tablespoon | 81 |
| Peanuts, salted | 1 ounce | 125 |
| Potato chips | 1 ounce (14 chips) | 285 |
| Pretzels | ½ ounce | 500 |
| Relish | 1 tablespoon | 95 |
| Soy sauce | 1 tablespoon | 1,099 |
| Tartar sauce | 1 tablespoon | 220 |
| Worcestershire sauce | 1 tablespoon | 165 |
| **Sweets** | | |
| Apple pie | 1 slice | 406 |
| Banana cream pie | 1 slice | 262 |
| Blueberry pie | 1 slice | 296 |
| Cherry pie | 1 slice | 401 |
| Chocolate bar | 2 ounces | 190 |
| Chocolate brownie with nuts | 1 medium | 126 |

| Food | Amount | Sodium (milligrams) |
| --- | --- | --- |
| Chocolate fudge | 1 piece (1″) | 86 |
| Chocolate syrup | 1 tablespoon | 10 |
| Doughnut | 1 medium | 165 |
| Lemon meringue pie | 1 slice | 338 |
| Pudding, chocolate | 1 cup | 139 |
| Pudding, tapioca | 1 cup | 390 |
| **Vegetables** | | |
| Artichoke | 1 medium | 30 |
| Asparagus | 8 spears | 6 |
| Beans, green | 1 cup | 3 |
| Beans, kidney | 1 cup | 5 |
| Beans, navy | 1 cup | 5 |
| Beet greens | 1 cup | 115 |
| Beets | 1 cup | 81 |
| Broccoli | 1 cup | 89 |
| Cabbage | 1 cup | 145 |
| Carrot | 1 medium | 34 |
| Cauliflower | 1 cup | 12 |
| Celery | 1 cup | 135 |
| Chickpeas | 1 cup | 22 |
| Corn, canned | 1 cup | 475 |
| Corn, fresh, on cob | 1 medium ear | 2 |
| Cucumber, fresh | 1 cup | 3 |
| Cucumber pickle | 1 cup | 1,425 |
| Lettuce, Bibb | 1 cup | 9 |
| Mushrooms, cooked | 1 cup | 960 |
| Olives, green | 1 cup | 850 |
| Onion | 1 cup | 14 |
| Peas, canned | 1 cup | 236 |
| Peas, fresh | 1 cup | 1 |
| Potato | 1 medium | 4 |
| Potato salad | 1 cup | 1,322 |

| Food | Amount | Sodium (milligrams) |
| --- | --- | --- |
| Potatoes, mashed, with butter and milk | 1 medium | 663 |
| Pumpkin | 1 cup | 5 |
| Radish | 1 medium | 1 |
| Sauerkraut | 1 cup | 1,755 |
| Spinach, canned | 1 cup | 400 |
| Spinach, fresh | 1 cup | 90 |
| Squash, acorn | 1 cup | 8 |
| Squash, butternut | 1 cup | 20 |
| Sweet potato | 1 medium | 20 |
| Tofu (bean curd) | 1 cup | 21 |
| Tomato, raw | 1 medium | 15 |
| Zucchini | 1 cup | 24 |

This table provides a good starter map of where the salt lies. If you're going to investigate the matter in further detail—and it's recommended that you do—most health product stores and booksellers carry pocket-sized handbooks listing the salt quotient of a large number of comestibles, both raw and commercially prepared. See, for example, *The Sodium Counter,* by Annette B. Natow and Jo-Ann Hesun, which gives the salt content of 9,000 foods. Take a look also at Kathy Stone's *Pocket Edition: Fat, Sodium, Cholesterol, and Calorie Counter*.

Once you're familiar with the general salt content in a variety of foods, you'll want to plan your daily menu to include plenty of low-sodium foods and a minimum of high-sodium ones. Shopping will temporarily take longer once you've decided to go no- or low-salt. But soon you'll have the new regimen down pat, and shopping for these items will become routine.

A few hints:

• Read the labels of all canned and packaged foods carefully. For most foods the salt content is listed on the side of the container. Keep the following salt content standards in mind. They were set by the Food and Drug Administration.

| | |
|---|---|
| NO SODIUM | Contains 5 mg or less sodium per serving. |
| VERY LOW SODIUM | Contains 34 mg or less sodium per serving. |
| LOW SODIUM | Contains 140 mg or less sodium per serving. |
| REDUCED SODIUM | The regular amount of sodium added to this food has been reduced by 75 percent. |
| UNSALTED | This product has been produced with no salt whatsoever. This label is used on foods that normally contain generous amounts of salt, such as butter, mayonnaise, ketchup, salad dressing, etc. |

• Note the listings of additives and preservatives on the side of bottles and cans. Avoid products that contain large quantities of sodium compound additives such as sodium benzoate, sodium nitrate, sodium nitrite, sodium sulfite, and so forth. Beware of MSG, baking powder, and baking soda.

• Consciously avoid reaching for high-salt "danger foods" from the supermarket shelf. These foods include potato chips, salted and buttered popcorn, creamed and canned vegetables, meat tenderizer, hot dogs, sausage, salted nuts and seeds, pretzels, dill pickles, enchilada dinners, frozen pizza, bread stuffing mix, packaged sliced luncheon meats, green olives, crystallized or glazed fruits (like maraschino cherries), sauerkraut, anchovies, bacon, herring, smoked or salted meats and fish, instant pudding mixes, chili sauce, steak sauce, soy sauce, and most brands of TV dinners (unless otherwise labeled).

• Low-sodium breakfast cereals include puffed rice, puffed wheat, shredded wheat, and cereals with "low salt" on the label. Many of the more nutritious breakfast cereals, such as granola, muesli, and instant oatmeal, are loaded with salt unless otherwise labeled.

• If you constantly feel the impulse to reach for high-salt foods while shopping, try avoiding those areas of the supermarket that display them. This is easier done than you might imagine, as most supermarkets are designed with the staples—fruits, vegetables, meat, dairy products, and bread—located on the four outer aisles of the store, forming a kind of square. Try sticking to these aisles as much as possible while you shop, journeying into the inner danger zones only when you must. If you go to market with another person, have him or her shop the inner aisles for you.

• Assume that canned and processed foods contain many salt-bearing additives plus high-salt extras like MSG. Avoid salty, heavily processed products, and reach for the fresh alternatives. Instead of buying creamed corn try the fresh variety. Instead of preserved canned ham cook a fresh ham at home. And note that tuna fish in water, though naturally high in salt content, contains less sodium than tuna packed in oil.

• When shopping at your local pharmacy read the labels on all medicines before purchasing. Many common over-the-counter items such as laxatives, aspirin, antacids, cough medicines, and sedatives contain large amounts of salt. So do many antibiotics. Ask your pharmacist if low-salt or no-salt versions of these products are available.

### 3. Using less salt at the table

First order of the day: Remove the saltshaker from the table before you sit down to eat. To paraphrase an old proverb, what the eye doesn't see the stomach doesn't yearn for.

Another trick is to give the saltshaker its honored place at the table but refill it with a salt substitute. There are a variety of these products available today at health food stores and in some supermarkets. Made from a medley of substances including seeds, dried vegetables, seaweed, herbs, and spices, these mixtures come reasonably close to approximating the taste of real salt.

One product worth investigating is Sea Seasoning's

Nori Granules with Ginger, which makes use of nori, a pressed seaweed (the kind used in Japanese restaurants for wrapping sushi), to give foods a pungent flavor. Walnut Acres markets a concoction called Vegetable Flakes that exploits the naturally salty taste of certain vegetables. Salt Sense, a Diamond Crystal product available at most supermarkets, contains 33 percent less sodium per spoonful than regular salt and is a good have-your-salt-and-eat-it-too compromise for people who don't want to cut back entirely. In some health food stores you'll also find a product known as go-maiso, a macrobiotic-inspired preparation of sea salt and sesame seeds. While not entirely salt free, this interesting blend cuts down dramatically on the amount of sodium you'll use at each serving, and tastes as good as or better than ordinary table salt in the bargain (followers of the macrobiotic system of eating claim that gomaiso is also useful for calming seasickness and relieving heartburn).

Or try making your own gomaiso:

Lightly and slowly brown 1 cup sesame seeds in a skillet over a low flame. Stir and shake the skillet while cooking to prevent the seeds from burning. When the seeds are brown, pour them into a bowl and mix in ½ teaspoon of sea salt. Grind the mixture with a mortar and pestle or in a blender until the seeds are fully crushed but not totally pulped. Then pour the mixture into a jar and keep it tightly closed. Use gomaiso exactly the same way you would use salt.

Other salt substitutes are similarly easy to prepare. Here's one to try.

Mix the following herbs and spices together in a bowl:

> 1 teaspoon sesame seeds
> 1 teaspoon finely ground black pepper
> 1 teaspoon garlic powder
> 1 teaspoon onion powder
> 1 teaspoon dried basil
> 1 teaspoon celery seed
> 1 teaspoon allspice
> 1 teaspoon mustard powder
> 1 teaspoon thyme
> 1 teaspoon oregano

Pour the mixture into a mortar or a blender and grind until the blend takes on a granular consistency. Pack the mixture into a saltshaker and use as desired.

Finally, consider stand-alone spices as prime enliveners of meats and vegetables. The following condiments are not salt substitutes exactly, in that they don't taste particularly salty. But they do impart their own savory and interesting flavors:

| | | |
|---|---|---|
| cloves | ginger | oregano |
| chili powder | marjoram | paprika |
| cumin | mustard, dry | sage |
| dill | nutmeg | tarragon |
| garlic powder | onion powder | thyme |

## 4. Using less salt when cooking

The aim here is to substantially reduce—or totally eliminate—salt from the cooking process.

This goal is best approached in stages. Here's how it works.

In the first two weeks reduce the amount of salt added to the foods you prepare by 25 percent.

The next two weeks cut the amount by 50 percent.

For dieters who prefer a low-salt (as opposed to a no-salt) diet, this is a good place to stop. A month has passed now, and your sodium intake is halved. Assuming you're salt-sensitive, you should see the positive effects register in your blood pressure.

Those who wish to go further and achieve a salt-free diet can cut salt usage back by 75 percent at the beginning of the fifth week, then eliminate it entirely at the end of the six week. By now your taste buds have been conditioned to demand less salt, so cutting the cord entirely should be easy.

A few cooking tricks of the trade always help the process along.

For example, in the beginning, especially during the second and third week of salt cutback, you'll find that your food tastes somewhat bland. As you and others at the table gradually get used to the new regimen, time will cure this problem on its own. In the meantime, help the situation along by availing yourself of the arsenal of food flavoring aids available to every cook: fruits, condiments, and dairy toppings, as well as herbs and spices.

For example, try adding basil and chives to scrambled eggs. Have your sunny-side eggs straight up with a tarragon topping. Garnish potatoes with olive oil, dill, and oregano. Add curry powder to vegetable mixtures. Add a quarter tablespoon of chili powder to a mixture of corn, tomatoes, and green peppers. Nutmeg is a natural boost to the taste of summer squash, as are pieces of chopped apple soaked in honey and cooked with the squash. Enliven pork dishes with garlic and sage, chicken dishes with paprika. Cover tomato slices with fresh basil leaves, scallions, and onion slices. Substitute fresh bean curd cubes for salty cheese in your salads. Add low-fat yogurt to meats and potatoes (among dairy products, yogurt is relatively low in sodium). Make pizza with vegetable toppings rather than sausage and cheese; try onions, peppers, broccoli. Garnish cooked carrots with poppy seeds and olive oil. Boiled cabbage comes alive with dill and caraway seeds. Ginger and scallions are an ideal topping for chicken dishes. Bring out the flavor of lamb by covering its skin with rosemary, thyme, and marjoram, and by inserting garlic buds into the skin before cooking.

Taste levels in low-salt and no-salt dishes can also be ratcheted up by using fresh fruits. Prunes and apricots work well in chicken dishes. Pineapple and orange slices are a perfect complement to roast chicken. Baked apple goes wonderfully with most meats. Applesauce is a natural when served with pork chops. Squeeze lemon juice onto your lamb roast before cooking. Use cranberry sauce with chicken and pork (not just turkey). Serve mint jelly on the side with lamb.

In other words, stretch yourself; be inventive. Take advantage of the tools you already have at hand. Herbs, spices, fruits, condiments, salt substitutes, juices (like lemon and orange), all can make a low-salt meal come alive.

You may wish to enlist one or two low-salt cookbooks as allies in this endeavor. Several excellent works are currently available. These include *No Salt, No Sugar, No Fat Cookbook,* by Jacqueline Williams and Goldie Silverman; *A Fare for the Heart: Cleveland Clinic Cookbook,* by Jacques Pepin; *American Heart Association Low-Salt Cookbook: A Complete Guide to Reducing Sodium and Fat in the Diet,* by Rodman D. Starke; and *Secrets of Salt-Free Cooking,* by Jeanne Jones.

Note that a full low-salt, antihypertensive menu is provided in Chapter 6 of this book.

# 5

## Things to Eat and Not Eat for Better Blood Pressure

### Eater Beware

The past decades have witnessed remarkable advances in nutritional awareness among Americans and within the health care profession. Fifty years ago the content and quality of the food we ate was largely ignored by health care professionals and the field of nutritional counseling was virtually nonexistent.

Today as never before we understand that we are what we eat, and that food can exert powerful and complex influences on the way we feel, how clearly we think, our energy level, the ups and downs of our emotional life, and even the number of years we live. The result of this new understanding has gone a long way toward raising national standards of health.

Of course, at one time or another all of us become careless eaters. We miss meals, drink too much alcohol, overeat, junk out on sugars and fats.

On a weekly or even monthly basis these slips don't amount to much. The digestive system is an amazingly resilient group of organs built to take a beating. Yet over the long haul, year after year, decade after decade, the consequences of poor nutritional habits add up, until eventually, like water wearing down a stone, the protective mechanisms that keep our organs finely tuned begin to erode. Result: disease. As the saying goes, "Health begins and ends in the stomach."

We've already seen the role that salt plays in generating hypertension. In this section we'll look at a number of other foods and drinks, both the helpful kinds and the harmful kinds, and discover how by using these foods wisely—or avoiding them entirely—we gain a powerful ally against the subtle wiles of hypertension.

## Things Not to Consume:
### Never, Sometimes, Perhaps

**Smoking**

Since we already know that smoking contributes to a variety of fatal cardiovascular disorders, it is perhaps redundant to call attention to its negative effects on blood pressure.

Yet at first glance smoking appears to be only a minor villain in the blood pressure picture. We know, for instance, that smoking a cigarette or inhaling the smoke from a pipe or cigar can immediately raise one's blood pressure by several points. The same is true when using "smokeless tobacco," i.e., chewing tobacco and snuff. A few minutes later, however, readings return to normal; the rise is only temporary. As yet there is not much evidence that smoking by itself is a seminal cause of hypertension.

Does this get smoking off the hook as a cardiovascular menace?

Certainly not. According to the American Heart Association and hundreds of other medical authorities, the single most important step you can take to insure the health of your heart is to *not smoke*. Period.

This means that while there may or may not be a one-on-one relationship between smoking and high blood pressure, inhaling tobacco smoke creates such havoc with the lungs, heart, stomach, and circulatory system, and promotes so many deadly diseases—stroke, cancer, emphysema, and heart attack among them—that the verdict is clearly in: If you have high blood pressure, don't smoke. If you have normal blood pressure, don't smoke. Whatever you do, don't smoke!

A number of stop-smoking programs, many of them free or inexpensive, exist today in communities around the country. Ask your doctor for a reference. Or get in touch with the local chapter of the American Lung Association or the American Heart Association for more information.

### Alcohol

After many years of clinical trials we now know that the excessive consumption of alcoholic beverages puts one at risk of increased blood pressure, and that people who are already hypertensive are especially vulnerable.

More significantly, for certain people alcohol elevates blood pressure *on its own*, independent of other causes (such as extra weight or poor diet). If you are sensitive in this way, all you need do is down three or four drinks and presto, your systolic blood pressure shoots up 4 or 5 points, your diastolic 2 or 3. It's been estimated that up to 5 percent of people with hypertension suffer from high blood pressure *strictly because of their drinking habits*. The ailment is known as *alcoholic hypertension*.

What exactly constitutes excessive drinking? While estimates differ, the following guidelines will serve:

- wine—more than 7 ounces a day
- beer—more than 24 ounces a day (there are 12 ounces in a can of beer)
- hard liquor *(whiskey, gin, vodka, rum, etc.)*—more than 2 ounces a day

Although only a small percentage of hypertensives suffer from alcoholic hypertension, there are secondary problems related to drinking that make it a danger to anyone with volatile blood pressure. Alcohol is high in empty calories, for instance, and for many drinkers these calories are quickly transformed into added weight. Extra poundage, we know, increases blood pressure.

Alcohol use often goes hand in hand with snacking— especially consuming salty snacks like peanuts, pretzels, and popcorn. If you're salt-sensitive, a bout of heavy drinking mixed with high salt intake can be disastrous to blood pressure readings

Note too that commercial alcoholic drinks are filled with salty additives. One can of beer contains preservatives, fermenting agents, artificial colorings, foam inhibitors, and more, many of which are laden with salt.

Alcohol, we also know, stimulates the hormone cortisol. Increased amounts of this chemical trigger salt retention and potassium loss in the body. Both are serious reactions for anyone suffering from hypertension.

Finally, note that alcohol intake, especially heavy alcohol intake, can in some cases interfere with the action of hypertensive medications (as well as other medications), producing alarming side effects. On rare occasions it can send a drinker to the hospital. Consult with your physician on this one.

Persons suffering from high blood pressure, in other words, are cautioned not to push the drinking envelope too far, and to keep their alcohol intake modest. This means no more than one or two drinks a day. For persons with serious hypertension, complete abstention is best.

## Caffeine

For years researchers have been trying to pin a variety of ailments on caffeine, a naturally occurring alkaloid found in cocoa, soft drinks, tea, and, most prominently, coffee. Since caffeine is a stimulant that increases heart rate and urine production (and in large doses produces insomnia, restlessness, heart irregularities, and even delirium), caffeine was one of the first food substances to be targeted by hypertension researchers. After all, they reasoned, the average American has a greater than 50 percent chance of dying from a heart attack, *and* the average American drinks at least three cups of coffee a day.

Attempts to convict caffeine of cardiovascular crimes have, however, met with mixed results.

Some years ago researchers at Duke University did discover that several cups of coffee a day appeared to raise the diastolic readings a few points in some people. This response, it turned out, was transient, and did not produce long-term changes. What's more, since the time of the Duke evaluation many other studies have been carried out to determine the effects of coffee on the heart and circulatory system, and to date the findings from these studies are conflicting at best.

One medical group in Canada, for example, examined the results of eleven worldwide studies of caffeine to test the oft-quoted wisdom that four cups of coffee a day increases risk of coronary heart disease. The verdict? According to these studies, people who drink four and even six cups of coffee a day develop coronary problems with more or less the same frequency as those who drink no coffee at all. These findings were seconded by a recent study done at Harvard University of forty-five thousand male coffee drinkers. Again, no evidence was found to show that drinking coffee, even in excessive amounts, contributes to heart disease.

What conclusion are we to draw from all this evidence?

The answer is that coffee is surely not the best item on the menu for you to take into your system, especially if you suffer from hypertension. A cup or two a day will probably not make much difference in your overall health, but it pays to be careful. Certainly any food that raises your blood pressure a notch or two, even for a short time, is something to be wary of. Note, incidentally, that studies done in Scandinavia suggest that coffee prepared by the boiling method raises cholesterol levels slightly, while filtered coffee has no effect on blood lipids.

### Cholesterol

Contrary to popular belief, cholesterol does not enter our bodies solely via animal foods such as eggs, meat, and dairy products. It is also manufactured inside the body itself, where it performs several critical jobs: the transportation of fats, the production of hormones and bile salts, and the formation of the fatty sheath that surrounds and protects the nerve cells.

But this important substance is beneficial to human health only up to a point. When the body's cholesterol reserves become too great, usually through an overabundance of high-cholesterol foods, deposits of cholesterol-laden plaque build up in the blood vessels. These deposits eventually become so large they cause the vessels to stiffen and narrow, producing resistance against the blood flow. This resistance causes the circulatory system to work harder and elevates blood pressure, putting a person at greater risk of heart disease, stroke, and atherosclerosis.

What constitutes a high cholesterol count?

A healthy adult should have a blood cholesterol level below 200 mg/dl (decaliter). Anything above that number ushers one into the risk zone. Some physicians even believe that for people who have one or more hypertension risks (family history, say, or overweight), a count of 180 mg/dl is preferable. Statistically, for every 1 percent reduction in the blood cholesterol level a person's chances of heart attack are reduced by 2 percent.

For purposes of nutrition, moreover, there are two different kinds of cholesterol, "good" cholesterol, known as *high-density lipoproteins* (or, more commonly, HDLs) and "bad" cholesterol, *low-density lipoproteins* (LDLs).

High measurements of LDL cholesterol participate in the buildup of plaque in the veins, contributing to the development of high blood pressure and atherosclerosis. According to the National Institutes of Health, the following guidelines should be heeded concerning LDL levels:

- desirable level—below 130 mg/dl
- borderline—130 to 160 mg/dl
- high-risk—over 160 mg/dl

HDLs, on the other hand, help lower the level of insoluble fats and cholesterol by removing them from the arteries and returning them to the liver for reprocessing. This recycling process prevents plaque buildup and protects the body against cardiovascular disease.

Though an acceptable level of HDLs for men is around 45 mg/dl, and for women around 55 mg/dl, HDLs are usually expressed as a ratio of total blood cholesterol. Besides showing the relationship of the good cholesterol to all other cholesterol in your body, this ratio is a predictor of risk for heart disease.

For example, a good ratio for a man is around 4; which means that if a man has a total cholesterol of 200 mg/dl, 50 mg/dl of this is in the form of HDLs.

For women a healthy ratio should be a bit lower. Around 2.3 to 4 is average; anything above 4.7 is high. A woman with a ratio of, say, 5 is at a considerably higher risk for cardiovascular disease than a woman with a ratio of 2.5.

How do we raise our HDL levels? Through regular exercise, weight control, stress control, and, once again, by carefully watching what we eat. All cholesterol comes from animal foods: meat and dairy. There is absolutely no cholesterol in plant foods: fruits, vegetables, grains. The following foods are all heavy in cholesterol:

| | | |
|---|---|---|
| beef | eggs | oysters |
| butter | ice cream | pork |
| cheese | lamb | pound cake |
| chicken | lard | shrimp |
| crab | milk, whole | squid |
| cream | organ meats (e.g., liver) | |

## Dietary Fats

As you can see from the above list, a number of cholesterol-laden foods come in the form of high-fat foods. But while they are often spoken of interchangeably, fats and cholesterol are different.

Cholesterol, as we've seen, is a protective substance produced naturally by the body—in the liver, to be exact. Dietary fats, on the other hand, are a basic nutrient, one of the three main food groups along with protein and carbohydrates. While cholesterol usually accompanies dietary fat, dietary fats do not always contain cholesterol.

For example, a three-and-a-half-ounce pork chop contains around 30 grams of fat and 80 milligrams of cholesterol. A tablespoonful of olive oil contains 10 grams of fat but *zero* milligrams of cholesterol. Moral: Don't automatically assume that every high-fat food is also a cholesterol carrier. It often is. But not always.

Note also that not all dietary fats are the same, and that basically they fall into two categories: animal fat and vegetable fat.

Animal fat reaches us via meat, saturated fats, dairy products, and eggs. Vegetable fats are derived from grains, fruits, seeds, vegetables, and legumes. While the issue is a complicated one, generally speaking, the foods that build cholesterol in our arteries and that add extra inches to our girth are also the ones that are heavy in animal fat. It is, therefore, animal fat that people with hypertension are well advised to monitor and control.

The following tips and suggestions will help you succeed at this task:

• If you eat meat, eat lean meat. Avoid eating too much pork and roast beef, and when you do, try shopping for the leaner varieties. Interestingly, dried beef and chipped beef contain a good deal less fat than unprocessed beef, but at the same time they are both alarmingly high in salt. Avoid them if possible. Instead, get in the habit of eating small quantities of chicken, fish, or turkey (nutritionists speak of serving meat portions the size of a deck of playing cards). They're leaner, cheaper, and can be made into an endless variety of tempting dishes.

• Make a concerted effort to limit the use of commercial foods that display a fat or oil first on the ingredients list on the side of the container. Fats to be especially wary of include:

| | |
|---|---|
| butter | palm oil |
| cocoa butter | vegetable shortening |
| coconut (and coconut oil) | whole-milk products |
| hydrogenated vegetable | (cream, cheese, |
| oil | yogurt, etc.) |

• Take a hint from Middle Eastern cuisine: Keep your meat portions small. Instead of eating three ounces of meat at a sitting, cut this amount in half. A little meat goes a long way, especially if the rest of the meal includes starches such as beans, bread, and potatoes.

• When making soup, use bouillon cubes instead of meat stock. Your soup won't have as much body this way, but you can compensate by adding hearty grains to the soup like rice or noodles.

• Once or twice a week try substituting vegetable protein for meat. Beans are an especially good meat surrogate. They are filling enough to be eaten as a main course and they are not fattening. Bean curd—tofu— also makes an excellent meat stand-in.

• Avoid fried foods, especially deep-fried foods. Bake, boil, barbecue, and broil instead. Also avoid using fats to flavor your vegetables. Try fresh herbs and spices instead.

• Use unsaturated vegetable oils such as canola, olive, safflower, corn, and soybean oil. When cooking with oil, use it sparingly. A drop or two in the bottom of the pan is fine for sautéing. When mixing salad dressings, use recipes that don't call for oil. An interesting oriental substitute for the oil-and-vinegar standby is made as follows:

> 1 tofu cake
> ¼ cup water
> 1 onion, chopped
> ½ teaspoon sesame oil
> Lemon juice

Mash the tofu and add the other ingredients. Stir the mixture until it reaches a creamy consistency. Use on any fresh green salad.

• When buying dairy products, go the low-fat or no-fat route: low-fat/no-fat cottage cheese, low-fat/no-fat milk, low-fat/no-fat sour cream, low-fat/no-fat yogurt, low-fat/no-fat cream cheese, and so forth. Skim milk and nonfat dry milk are also good, though be warned of their rather high salt content. If you haven't tried buttermilk for a while, you may be pleasantly surprised. Despite the "butter" in its name, buttermilk tends to be relatively low in fat and makes a hearty thirst-quencher.

• Stick to low-fat desserts. Fruits are perfect. Stay away from cakes, ice cream, cookies, pies. They are all primary cholesterol offenders. If you do choose to indulge yourself, stick with the low-fat cakes, cookies, and so forth.

• Limit your egg intake. The yolk is high in cholesterol. Keep your egg count at two or three eggs a week.

• Reduce your dietary fat intake and you'll automatically reduce your cholesterol intake, especially when you cut down on animal fats. Include no more than 20 percent fats in your diet. The other 80 percent should come from protein and carbohydrates. And try to take in less than 300 milligrams of cholesterol per day.

### Licorice

Medicinally, licorice is thought by many herbalists to be an immune system booster, and is believed to have anti-inflammatory and antitumor effects. For candy lovers it makes a delicious confection. In Chinese medicine it is the most widely used of all herbs.

But for those who suffer from hypertension (or from kidney or heart problems), licorice is red-flagged. In certain people it increases the formation of a hormone known as aldosterone, which encourages the body to retain salt. Elevated blood pressure can result.

If you are a licorice addict and if you are loath to give up this gummy treat entirely, it's best to keep your consumption modest.

## Foods That Help

Just as there are foods that contribute to increased blood pressure, so there are foods that help keep blood pressure under control. Pay particular attention to the dietary factors discussed below, and try to incorporate the appropriate foods into your diet whenever you can.

### Minerals

#### 1. Potassium

Potassium has a diuretic effect on the body's fluid levels. When adequate amounts of this mineral are present in the body, they help the excretion of salt and keep sodium levels in balance. Too little potassium promotes excess water retention, which in turn leads to salt retention and elevated pressures. The blood pressure of people who favor a high-potassium diet, or who take potassium supplements, tends to be lower than that of people who lack this mineral in their diet.

How much potassium should a person with hypertension take every day?

Approximately 5,500 milligrams daily is adequate. This is a figure many times above the minimum RDA for people with normal blood pressure (775 milligrams).

If you are on a diuretic medication for hypertension, moreover, or if you are taking corticosteroid drugs, you may need even larger amounts, as both types of medication (especially diuretics) leach large quantities of potassium out of the body. It's also wise to be careful of laxative drugs, heavy alcohol intake, and profuse sweating, all of which wash away stores of precious minerals.

Potassium deficiency, known as *hypokalemia*, can be recognized from such symptoms as fatigue, dizziness, muscle weakness, and sleepiness (as well as heart irregularities and muscle paralysis in severe cases). If you have a tendency toward high blood pressure and also suffer from any chronic digestive tract disorder such as gastroenteritis, be especially concerned: frequent vomiting and diarrhea generate potassium loss through the excretion of potassium-rich gastrointestinal fluids.

What's the best way to get your daily quota of potassium?

Potassium supplements are useful and accessible at any health products stores. Potassium reserves can also be bolstered in a natural way by means of your diet. For example, a 1992 study published in the *Journal of the American Medical Association* showed that eating increased amounts of potassium-bearing foods substantially reduces the need for blood pressure medication for some people. Other studies have proved potassium's dietary usefulness as well.

Though potassium is found in almost everything we eat, it is especially prevalent in fruits, beans, fish, meat, seeds, and whole grains. Anyone with irregular blood pressure is well advised to include six or seven of the high-potassium foods shown in Table 6 in his or her diet every day.

### Table 6: High-Potassium Foods

| Food | Amount | Potassium (milligrams) |
| --- | --- | --- |
| Apricots | 3 medium | 313 |
| Avocado | ½ | 680 |
| Banana | 1 medium | 451 |
| Beans, green | 3½ ounces | 260 |
| Bran, wheat | 3½ ounces | 1,121 |
| Bread, whole wheat | 3½ ounces | 273 |
| Broccoli | 1 cup | 235 |
| Cantaloupe | ½ medium | 812 |
| Chicken | 6 ounces | 401 |
| Flounder | 6 ounces | 585 |
| Lettuce | 3½ ounces | 264 |
| Orange juice | 3½ ounces | 200 |
| Peanuts | ½ cup | 709 |
| Peas, raw | 3½ ounces | 316 |
| Pecans | ½ cup | 333 |
| Pork, fat trimmed | 6 ounces | 533 |
| Potato, baked | 1 medium | 610 |
| Raisins | ½ cup | 545 |
| Salmon | 6 ounces | 761 |
| Sunflower seeds | ½ cup | 420 |
| Sweet potato | 1 medium | 397 |
| Tomato | 1 medium | 254 |
| Tuna | 6 ounces | 578 |
| Turkey | 6 ounces | 549 |

## 2. Calcium

A 1998 article in *The New York Times* announced that "calcium is fast emerging as the nutrient of the decade, a substance with such diverse roles in the body that virtually no major organ system escapes its influence." There is a large amount of clinical research to back that statement up.

Recent studies published in the *British Medical Journal*, for example, show that women who take calcium supplements during pregnancy bear children with lower-than-average blood pressures. In an issue of the *American Journal of Clinical Nutrition*, it was reported that a research team at the University of Southern California discovered that by adding calcium to the diet of teenagers, who typically eat a low-calcium diet, the subjects' average blood pressure became consistently lower. Still another study showed that people who add 1,000 milligrams a day of calcium to their diet experience measurably lower blood pressure readings.

There are many similar studies.

But is it this simple? Just increase calcium intake and your blood pressure goes down?

Not necessarily. Other studies show no correlation between calcium use and hypertension control. Some researchers believe that calcium helps regulate blood pressure, but only in people who are salt-sensitive.

One double-blind crossover study, for example, took twenty-three subjects who were salt-sensitive and twenty-three who were not. All subjects were given 1.5 grams of calcium carbonate a day for eight weeks. At the end of this period, the study showed that calcium supplementation produced effective blood pressure reduction in salt-sensitive persons but *not* in non-salt-sensitive persons.

What's the verdict?

The verdict is that there is basically more than enough evidence to suggest that calcium does play some role in blood pressure regulation, and that taking extra amounts can help. The worst-case scenario is that it *won't* lower your blood pressure. No harm done. And the added calcium may well provide you with other benefits, such as help with osteoporosis. The minimum RDA for calcium is 800 to 1,000 milligrams a day, and a bit more for people with hypertension.

The foods that contain the highest amounts of calcium are dairy products: cheese, milk, cream, yogurt, buttermilk, butter. These foods also tend to be high in both salt and cholesterol. But there's a way around that problem. By being clever in your menu planning, you can get all the calcium you need and at the same time keep your salt and cholesterol intake to a reasonable level. Try the following tricks:

• Eat lots of nonfat yogurt. This tasty food is loaded with calcium. But unlike most dairy products, it's low in salt. For example, a cup of yogurt carries 300 milligrams of calcium and only 128 milligrams of salt. An added benefit is that you receive large stores of potassium—358 milligrams per cup, to be exact. Add bananas, almonds, dates, or wheat germ to your yogurt and you'll get lots more.

• Be aware that vitamin D's primary function in the body is to regulate calcium. This important nutrient ensures that special cells in the small intestine absorb calcium; it maintains adequate calcium levels in the bloodstream; it oversees the deposition of calcium into the teeth and bones; and it prevents needed stores of calcium from being excreted in the urine. One way to ensure an adequate amount of vitamin D in your diet is to take a good multivitamin that contains the required RDA of vitamin D (400 IU for children, 200 IU for adults), and to eat a vitamin D–rich diet. Foods with the highest vitamin D content include cod liver oil, salmon, mackerel, herring, and the grand winner, sardines, with approximately 1,500 IU per 3½ ounces. Lesser amounts of vitamin D are found in yogurt, butter, egg yolks, and liver, plus vitamin D–enriched milk and breakfast cereals. Exposure to sunlight helps the body produce its own vitamin D.

• Become familiar with the calcium content of *non-dairy* foods and add these foods to your diet. There are a number of fruits and vegetables in this category you might not think of as high-calcium bearers. Dates, figs, and broccoli, for instance, deliver substantial amounts of this important mineral, and there are lots more. Table 7 provides a starter list.

### Table 7: Nondairy Calcium-Rich Foods

| Food | Amount | Calcium (milligrams) |
| --- | --- | --- |
| Almonds | 1 cup | 329 |
| Blackstrap molasses | 1 tablespoon | 145 |
| Brazil nuts, unsalted | 1 cup | 558 |
| Broccoli | 1 cup | 134 |
| Clams, steamed | 1 pound | 248 |
| Collards | 1 cup | 220 |
| Cream of Wheat | 1 cup | 99 |
| Dandelion greens | 1 cup | 252 |
| Dates | 1 cup | 220 |
| Farina | 1 cup | 183 |
| Figs | 1 cup | 320 |
| Kale, cooked | 1 cup | 230 |
| Lima beans | 1 cup | 91 |
| Mustard greens | 1 cup | 202 |
| Orange | 1 medium | 75 |
| Peanuts, unsalted | 1 cup | 173 |
| Salmon, canned | 1 pound | 888 |
| Sesame seeds | 1 cup | 253 |
| Soybeans, cooked | 1 cup | 146 |
| Tofu (bean curd) | 6 ounces | 175 |
| Turnip greens | 1 cup | 267 |

• If you check the list above you'll see that a pound of salmon alone provides nearly all of a person's daily requirement of calcium. Salmon is a kind of wonder food for the heart, with fish oils that are high in omega-3 fatty acids (more on this below). A three-ounce slice of salmon supplies you with lots of $B_{12}$ and at least 300 milligrams of potassium. Salmon is also a gourmet dish. Yet it's not a great deal more expensive than other fish.

• Add seaweed to your diet. Sea vegetables such as agar-agar, wakame, nori, and others contain more calcium than any other food outside the dairy kingdom. A cup of kelp delivers 1,670 milligrams of calcium. That's much more calcium than you'll find in a cup of milk, and *six times* more than in a cup of cottage cheese. The same serving of kelp brings you 11,000 milligrams of potassium, more potassium than you'll find in almost any other food in the world. Amazing! There's only one hitch: coming from the ocean, seaweeds are extremely salty. One way around this problem is to boil sea vegetables for five minutes, pour off the salty broth, add fresh water, then boil again for another few minutes. Repeat this process several times. Another trick is to serve and eat sea vegetables in small quantities. As you can see, a little seaweed goes a long way nutritionally.

## 3. Magnesium

While there is no conclusive evidence that extra magnesium lowers blood pressure, it is known that this critical mineral produces a relaxing effect on the blood vessels, preventing spasms and vessel constriction, and thus most likely affects the ups and downs of both the systolic and diastolic pressures. It has been observed in many studies that people with low levels of magnesium in their blood tend to have high blood pressure. It has also been shown that when magnesium supplements (or a magnesium-rich diet) are used to boost these levels, blood pressures drop.

Physiologically, magnesium works in direct partnership with calcium, relaxing the body's long strands of muscle (while calcium stimulates them), and helping constrict and relax the blood vessels. When the equilibrium between these two minerals is disrupted—too much magnesium and too little calcium, or vice versa—major problems can occur in the cardiovascular system, the nervous system, and the musculoskeletal structure.

For this reason magnesium and calcium are often blended together in the same supplement to provide a proper magnesium-calcium balance. Many people find these supplements useful, not only for blood pressure control but as an overall health booster and cardiovascular aid (people with heart trouble and those who have recently experienced heart attacks often show low levels of magnesium in their blood).

As far as food on the table is concerned, magnesium is present in a variety of common comestibles, including nuts, starchy fruits, dried legumes, cereals, soybeans, and dark leafy vegetables. Foods that are especially magnesium-rich include:

| | | |
|---|---|---|
| almonds | collard greens | shredded wheat |
| avocados | kidney beans | spinach |
| bananas | lima beans | Swiss chard |
| beet greens | milk, nonfat | tofu |
| brazil nuts | oatmeal | wheat germ |
| bread, whole wheat | peanuts | |
| cashews | peas | |
| | potato, baked | |

While clinical deficiencies of magnesium are unusual, many people remain on the margin without knowing it, taking in just enough magnesium to survive but not enough to stay healthy. For some people, especially those with hypertension, it is suspected that the standard RDA of 200 to 350 milligrams a day is not adequate, and that 400 or more milligrams a day is required for magnesium to do its proper work.

What causes magnesium depletion?

Both physical and environmental factors. Some people don't eat enough of the right mineral-laden foods. This is especially true for overly busy people who fail to watch their diet, and for those who eat too many high-calorie, low-nutrition junk foods. Mineral loss is also triggered by physiological distress. Prolonged gastrointestinal problems, for example, especially when accompanied by chronic diarrhea, can cause magnesium loss. So can lifestyle factors such as heavy drinking, personal trauma, and prolonged emotional upset. If you are currently under heavy psychological pressure, or if you are suffering from an emotional shock of any kind, be sure that your daily intake of potassium, magnesium, and calcium is adequate.

Note, finally, that some hypertension drugs, especially those in the diuretic family, deplete the body of its mineral stores—potassium, calcium, magnesium. If not compensated for, this depletion can exert harmful effects on blood pressure—all the more reason for persons with hypertension to eat a diet rich in the minerals discussed above.

**Further Dietary Aids**

### Fiber

During the 1970s British physicians Dr. Denis Burkitt and Dr. Hugh Trowell made a startling observation, based to a large extent on Burkitt's experience as a field doctor in Uganda. They observed that while certain intestinal ailments, such as cancer of the colon and diverticulosis (a chronic inflammation of the colon), have increased dramatically in the West over the past sixty or seventy years—a time span that coincides with the arrival of large-scale food-processing techniques—these degenerative diseases that so bedevil Western countries are still minimal in underdeveloped countries where food processing is rare.

Conclusion: A major reason for the high incidence of chronic degenerative diseases in the industrialized countries is that people who live there do not eat enough unprocessed fruits and vegetables, all of which are loaded with dietary fiber.

What is fiber exactly, and what value might it have for lowering blood pressure?

Fiber is the part of plant tissue that is not metabolized—the residue that passes through the body undigested and then exits largely intact. Fiber originates primarily from the cell walls of plants, where it serves to contain the cellular protoplasm that supports the plant's form and shape.

The primary benefit of a diet high in fiber is the strong absorbent action fiber exerts on the intestinal tract, drawing local stores of water into the feces and expanding their size and weight. This increased bulk allows the stool to transit more swiftly through the gut. People who eat high-fiber diets, tests show, eliminate more frequently, and void larger amounts of waste at each bowel movement.

Now it is known that the more quickly food transits the digestive system the less opportunity there is for bile salts from the liver to be reabsorbed back through the intestinal wall. These bile salts carry a great deal of cholesterol, and fiber is known to have a binding effect on these salts, causing them to "stick" to the fiber, become absorbed into it, and make a quick exit via elimination.

Lowering the intestinal reabsorption of bile salts, therefore, causes less plaque-building cholesterol to be deposited in the arteries. This in turn reduces the chances of blockage in the veins, and keeps blood flow resistance at a lower level. Countries in which the diet is high in fiber almost invariably have lower rates of hypertension and atherosclerosis than the industrialized countries.

An ancillary benefit of fiber is that it encourages weight loss, another antihypertension plus. Still other dividends include protection against diabetes, hemorrhoids, constipation, colon cancer, diverticulosis, and gallstones.

Quite a list.

Moral: If you suffer from hypertension, high-fiber foods are an easy and delicious way of helping your overall health. Table 8 provides a sampling of the fiber content in common foods.

**Table 8: Fiber Content in Common Foods**

| Food | Amount | Total dietary fiber (grams) |
|------|--------|-----------------------------|
| Apple | 1 whole | 3.0 |
| Asparagus | 4 spears | .9 |
| Avocado | 1 | 4.4 |
| Banana | 1 medium | 1.8 |
| Beans, green | 1 cup | 3.9 |
| Beets | 1 cup | 4.2 |
| Bran, wheat | 1 cup | 23.0 |
| Bread, pumpernickel | 1 slice | 1.2 |
| Bread, whole wheat | 1 slice | 2.4 |
| Broccoli | 1 cup | 2.2 |
| Carrot | 1 cup | 2.1 |
| Corn | 1 medium ear | 5.9 |
| Fig | 1 medium | 2.4 |
| Grits | ½ cup | 9.1 |
| Kidney beans | 1 cup | 2.0 |
| Lentil soup | 1 cup | 5.5 |
| Lettuce | 1 serving | 1.5 |
| Mango | 1 medium | 3.0 |
| Okra | 1 cup | 2.6 |
| Orange | 1 medium | 2.5 |
| Parsnip | 1 cup | 6.2 |
| Peach | 1 medium | 1.4 |
| Pear | 1 medium | 2.6 |
| Peas | 1 cup | 7.9 |
| Pineapple | 1 cup | 2.2 |
| Potato, baked in skin | 1 medium | 3.0 |
| Prunes | 5 medium | 5.0 |
| Raisins | 2 tablespoons | 1.2 |
| Rice, brown | 1 cup | 1.1 |
| Rice, white | 1 cup | 0.4 |
| Rolled oats | ½ cup | 4.5 |
| Spinach | 1 cup | 11.4 |
| Strawberries | 1 cup | 3.4 |
| Tomato | 1 medium | 2.1 |

**Fish and fish oils**

Findings from the two-year study widely known as DART (Diet and Reinfarction Trial) provide evidence that men who eat fish on a regular basis have approximately a 30 percent lower chance of heart attacks than those who seldom or never eat fish. Several other studies back up these trials. Eating fish just twice a week has also been found to reduce the risk of heart attack by as much as 25 to 50 percent.

The problem is that not all fish produce these effects.

Many standard chafing dish specials such as cod and flounder, for example, are of limited help in the blood pressure department. Same with shellfish and deep sea creatures. On the other hand, mackerel, sardines, tuna, shark, whitefish, bluefish, squid, and halibut are all believed to exert a strong positive effect on blood pressure, and to lower blood cholesterol levels as well.

Why these fish in particular?

Most likely because they are rich in omega-3 fatty acids, natural substances found in fish oil that appear to be effective in lowering blood pressure for people with mild hypertension, especially men. As of 1997 more than sixty double-blind studies have demonstrated that fish oil helps reduce blood pressure and lower cholesterol, sometimes to impressive degrees. (Flaxseed oil, whose active ingredient is alpha-linolenic acid, is sometimes taken in place of fish oil, and appears to be equally effective.)

But be warned: Fish oil is by no means a panacea for hypertension. Some studies are inconclusive; others cast doubt, while a few suggest that too much fish oil can actually *increase* the chance of coronary problems. Taken in large quantities, what's more, fish-oil supplements thin the blood to a risky degree, interfering with natural clotting mechanisms. Many doctors still consider the claims made for fish-oil supplements to be trendy at best.

All things considered, however, eating fish several times a week is clearly a healthy alternative, and taking modest amounts of fish-oil supplements once a day is helpful at best and harmless at worst. Like so many other possible but unproven hypertension remedies, these products may work for you, or they may not; but there's no harm in trying.

### Vitamins

While there is little evidence that any one particular vitamin helps decrease blood pressure, we do know that certain vitamins help cardiovascular health in general, and as far as hypertension goes that's a plus.

For instance, taking 1,000 milligrams of vitamin C every day for an extended period can help lower blood cholesterol by as much as 7 to 10 percent.

Several major studies demonstrate that because of its antioxidant properties, vitamin E helps prevent coronary disease and keeps the heart's pumping mechanism in good order. Though some controversy surrounds the question of vitamin E and the heart, the latest medical thinking, based on recent tests, is that taking 100 to 400 IU of vitamin E a day helps your heart in several basic ways, and that your circulatory system is aided too.

Finally, in instances where a person has recently suffered a heart attack, vitamin $B_3$, better known as niacin, can speed recovery and help prevent reoccurrence. Several major studies demonstrate that a daily dose of 1,500 milligrams of niacin a day lowers blood cholesterol and raises the "good" HDLs.

All in all, vitamins appear in some cases to be of benefit for the circulation in general—especially the vitamins listed above. Several other vitamins have been nominated as cardiovascular aids, vitamin D, folic acid, and beta-carotene, among them, but the evidence for these claims so far is unconvincing. The best strategy here is simply to make sure that you eat a nutrient-rich diet, that you avoid vitamin-depleting habits such as smoking, drinking, and drug taking, and that you take a good vitamin supplement once a day.

## Garlic

In the 1920s, articles were already appearing in medical magazines to the effect that garlic exerts a hypotensive—the opposite of hypertensive—effect on human beings and that it is useful both in lowering blood pressure and improving overall cardiovascular health. Recently, after an evaluation of sixteen clinical trials, it was shown that subjects who take the equivalent of one garlic clove a day experience a 12 percent reduction in total cholesterol levels. Garlic's effectiveness as a blood platelet thinner is also well known, and health care professionals recommend it along with aspirin for this purpose. In certain laboratory tests, garlic has been shown to reduce both systolic and diastolic pressures in human beings, sometimes to a substantial degree.

Certainly there is no hardship in eating a clove or two of this pungently delicious food every day. Do be aware though that cooking strips garlic of some medicinal benefits, and that for purposes of health raw garlic is the food of choice. If you are afraid of smelling too much like a garlic press, odor-free garlic capsules are available at any health supply store.

### Celery

Several years ago, as reported in *The New York Times*, the father of a medical student named Quant T. Le was diagnosed as having hypertension. Instead of beginning a regimen of antihypertensive medication, the elder Mr. Le availed himself of an ancient oriental remedy: he ate a quarter pound of celery every day for one week. At the end of this time his blood pressure had gone from 158 over 96 to 118 over 82.

This remarkable recovery intrigued young Quant T. Le so much that he and a doctor named William Elliot at the University of Chicago Medical Center began studying the chemical properties of celery. They soon discovered what they believed to be the ingredient responsible for Mr. Le senior's blood pressure drop: *3-n-butyl phthalide*. This chemical substance appears to relax the smooth muscles that line the blood vessels and to reduce the amount of catecholamines, or "fight-or-flight" hormones, in the bloodstream, which when roused constrict blood vessels and set off a chain reaction that ends with a rise in blood pressure.

Experimenting, the two doctors discovered that 3-n-butyl phthalide lowers blood pressure in rats by 14 percent. As a bonus, they found that it reduces blood cholesterol counts in human beings by approximately 7 percent. All this from eating four medium-sized stalks of celery a day.

As yet there have been few follow-up studies, and the celery cure remains anecdotal. But eating celery as a snack or with lunch and dinner is certainly a painless option. Try this experiment: Take your blood pressure, then eat four or five medium-sized stalks a day for two weeks, then take your blood pressure again and compare. Who knows?

# 6

## The All-Round Anti-hypertension Diet—A 30-Day Menu Planner with Recipes

### Summing Up

We've covered a lot of ground so far in part 3, on hypertension and diet. We've seen how important nutrients can be in affecting the ups and downs of blood pressure. Now let's review the most important food issues we've talked about, take a look at one version of an ideal hypertension diet, then put it all together in a day-to-day eating regimen that you can start using immediately, and that will play a substantial part in your efforts to bring your blood pressure permanently into the safety zone.

To summarize the important points made so far:

1. Salt intake can be a major factor in raising blood pressure, but only if a person is salt-sensitive. We receive dietary salt from five main sources: in our drinking water, in our food, salt that is added at the table, salt that is added during cooking, and salt that is present in food additives. With judicious cooking and eating habits, these sources can all be monitored and controlled.

2. In a sizable percentage of individuals, alcohol abuse raises blood pressure. In people who are not alcohol-sensitive but who drink heavily, alcohol can contribute to chronic hypertension over an extended period of time. Cigarettes raise blood pressure too, but only temporarily, and only a small amount. Nonetheless, the damage tobacco does to the lungs, heart, and circulatory system makes it cardiovascular enemy number one.

3. Caffeine exerts a minimal short-term effect on blood pressure, and is probably okay to ingest in small amounts. But do keep your caffeine intake modest. Caffeine is found in tea, cocoa, soft drinks, and, most of all, in coffee.

4. Strive to maintain a cholesterol level below 200. Do this by eating sensibly, avoiding a high-cholesterol, high-fat diet, shopping and preparing food wisely, using low-fat/no-fat products, and acquainting yourself with the cholesterol and fat count of the foods you most commonly eat.

5. Potassium, calcium, and magnesium all play key roles in keeping blood pressure at an even keel. Make sure you receive adequate supplies. If you use a calcium supplement, it's a good idea to take magnesium with it to maintain the proper calcium-magnesium balance. Most foods contain some potassium, and potassium deficiency is rare. Still, some people experience blood pressure reduction by taking potassium supplements. Experiment on your own.

6. A diet high in fiber is highly recommended for anyone suffering from hypertension. Fiber reduces blood cholesterol, speeds elimination, and aids digestion. Us-

ing the table provided in the fiber section on page 189, learn which foods are high in this important component and make sure your diet contains plenty of them.

7. There is strong, though not conclusive evidence to suggest that eating fish twice a week or taking omega-3 fish oil supplements helps reduce blood pressure. Mackerel, sardines, tuna, shark, whitefish, bluefish, and halibut are the best bets for this purpose. Flaxseed oil supplements are sometimes taken in place of fish oil.

8. While no single vitamin lowers blood pressure, vitamins C, E, and $B_3$ are important nutrients for the cardiovascular system, and anyone concerned with circulatory health should take them in liberal amounts every day. Claims have also been made for other vitamins—e.g., vitamin A and folic acid—but so far there is little clinical evidence to suggest that they affect blood pressure in any significant way.

## What Is the Best Diet for Hypertension?

Taking all the above points and including them as part of our meal-planning strategy, we can now ask the vital question: What is the best diet for people who suffer from chronic hypertension?

In 1994 a research study titled "Dietary Approaches to Stop Hypertension," or DASH, as it is now known, was carried out on 459 adult men and women by the National Heart, Lung and Blood Institute at four major clinical centers across the country. The test was designed to determine whether blood pressure can be reduced by a diet based on whole foods rather than individual nutrients.

The study focused on "high normal" and "mild" high blood pressure, that is, on people with systolic readings below 160 mm Hg and diastolic readings between 80 and 95 mm Hg.

Participants were assigned one of three diets to follow for eight weeks. These were:

1. A control diet made up of the types of food most Americans eat: low in vegetables and fruit, high in fat,

2. A diet similar to the above control diet but rich in fruits and vegetables,

3. A combination diet rich in vegetables, fruits, and low-fat dairy products, and with reduced saturated fat and total fat adding up to 27 percent of total caloric intake.

The result?

Those in the control group (no. 1) and those who ate the fruit-and-vegetable-rich diets (no. 2) showed few significant changes in blood pressure. Test subjects who ate the "combination" diet (no. 3) experienced average blood pressure drops of 5.5 points systolic and 3 points diastolic. Those with mild hypertension who ate the combination diet showed blood pressure drops of an average 11 points systolic and 5.5 points diastolic.

Clearly the DASH diet works. And clearly people who are serious about taming their blood pressure the natural way should give it a try. Here's a breakdown of how it works:

## The DASH Diet at a Glance

| Foods | Servings |
|---|---|
| 1. Dieters should eat 4 to 5 servings a day of **fruits**. | Typical fruit servings include a 6-ounce glass of fruit juice, ½ cup of fresh fruit, and 1 medium-sized fruit such as an apple or pear. |
| 2. Dieters should eat 2 to 3 cups a day of **low-fat dairy foods**. | Low-fat dairy food servings include an 8-ounce glass of low-fat milk, 1.5 ounces of low-fat cheese, and 1 cup of low-fat yogurt. |
| 3. Dieters should eat 4 to 5 servings a day of **vegetables**. | Typical vegetable servings include ½ cup of cooked vegetables such as beets or carrots, 1 cup of raw leafy vegetables, a 6-ounce glass of vegetable juice, one full-sized salad, and a crudités serving of 3 carrot stalks and 3 celery stalks. |
| 4. Dieters should eat 2 or less servings of **meat, poultry, and fish**. | Typical meat, poultry, and fish servings include 3 ounces of cooked fish, poultry, or red meat. |
| 5. Dieters should eat 4 to 5 servings a week of **nuts, seeds, and legumes**. | Typical nut, seed, and legume servings include 2 tablespoons of seeds, ½ cup of cooked legumes such as beans or peas, and ⅓ cup of nuts. |
| 6. Dieters should eat 7 to 8 servings a day of **grains and grain products**. | Typical grain servings include 1 slice of bread, a bagel or roll, ½ cup dried cereal, ½ cup of cooked pasta, and ½ cup of cooked rice, corn, barley, millet, or other grain. |

While the DASH diet is based on 2,000 calories a day, dieters who require a larger caloric intake increase their number of daily servings from a particular food group according to need.

DASH dieters are also exhorted to lower fat intake and to build meals around rice, beans, pasta, and vegetables rather than meat. When meat is eaten at all it should be the lean variety, and small portions are recommended. DASH dieters should be sparing of oils, and when using salad dressing should make it nonfat or low-fat.

Why does this diet work so well?

Dr. Frank Sacks, a professor of nutrition at the Harvard School of Public Health, helped set up the study. In July 1998 he told *The New York Times*: "I think the high potassium content of the diet pretty much explains why it lowers blood pressure. It's half or more of the effect. . . . Potassium might foster sodium excretion from the body. . . . Potassium seems much more effective in people who have more sodium in their diet."

According to Dr. Sacks, calcium and magnesium also probably play a role in making this diet—which is so heavy in fruits, vegetables, grains, and milk—effective.

## The 30-Day Antihypertension Diet

The following food regimen is based on the DASH specifications and fits all food serving categories given above.

The series of menus provides a balanced diet that is

low in salt, low in fat and cholesterol, rich in "heart-friendly" foods, easy to prepare, and effective for fighting hypertension.

Try it for the recommended period of time and see. Over the past few years thousands of men and women with mild to moderate hypertension have found that this tasty and easy-to-follow diet helps. Most likely it will help you too.

## Day One

Breakfast
Fruit juice of choice
Oatmeal with sliced banana and low-fat milk
Whole grain toast, 1 slice, with jelly or jam
Regular or herbal tea

Lunch
Mixed salad: chickpeas, carrots, cabbage, kidney beans,
    and tomato slices
Low-fat cottage cheese, 1 scoop
Whole grain bread, 1 slice
Fresh pineapple chunks

Dinner
Indian Vegetable Curry
Rice
Cold no-fat yogurt with sliced cucumber
Pita bread or Indian chapati, 2
Fruit salad

Snack
Fruit smoothie made with nonfat milk and fruit

## Indian Vegetable Curry

| | |
|---|---|
| 2 onions, chopped | Garlic powder, to taste |
| 2 tablespoons olive oil | Ginger, to taste |
| 1 tablespoon turmeric | 1 cup chopped carrots |
| ½ tablespoon curry powder | 1 cup fresh peas |
| Chili powder, to taste | 1 tablespoon lemon juice |

In a saucepan, fry the onions in the olive oil until they become transparent. Then add the turmeric and other seasonings. Add the carrots and sauté for several minutes.

Cover saucepan and cook another 15 minutes, then add the peas. Mix well, cover, and cook until the peas and carrots are dry and tender. Add the lemon juice a few minutes before the vegetables are ready. Pour the curry over rice and serve.

## Day Two

Breakfast
Fruit juice of choice
Shredded wheat with apple and banana slices and
  almonds
Whole grain toast, 1 slice, with low-fat spread
Regular or herbal tea

Lunch
Crudités: sliced celery, carrots, cucumber, and radish
Low-fat cottage cheese, 1 scoop, with fresh fruit of
  choice, sliced
Whole grain bread, 2 slices, with low-fat spread

Dinner
Vegetable Soup
Baked potato with low-fat sour cream
Spinach
Broiled halibut
Low-fat yogurt, 1 bowl, with hulled sunflower seeds

Snack
Fresh fruit of choice: apples, pears, etc.
Bread, 1 slice, with honey

## Vegetable Soup

¼ cup dried pinto beans
¼ cup lentils
¼ cup chopped carrots
¼ cup chopped celery
¼ cup barley
¼ cup green beans

1 chopped tomato
1 clove garlic
1 onion, chopped
1 teaspoon salt substitute
3 tablespoons safflower oil

Soak the pinto beans and lentils overnight. Drain. Fill a pot with 6 cups of water. Add the beans and lentils and cook until they're soft. Add the carrots, celery, barley, green beans, tomato, garlic, and onion, and simmer for 45 minutes. Add the salt substitute and oil, and cook for another several minutes.

## Day Three

Breakfast
Fruit juice of choice
Soft-boiled eggs, 2, sprinkled with bread crumbs
Fresh apple
Whole grain toast, 1 slice, with spread of choice
Regular or herbal tea

Lunch
Baked potato
Low-fat cottage cheese, 1 scoop, with banana and apple
  slices
Whole grain bread, 1 slice, with low-fat spread of choice

Dinner
Fresh salad: a variety of lettuces and other vegetables
Spinach Pie
Steamed, sliced beets
Bread of choice, 2 slices, with low-fat spread
Low-fat ice cream with fruit topping

Snack
Mix of almonds, walnuts, and pecans

## Spinach Pie

Pie pastry to line bottom of
   9-inch pan (your own or
   prepared)
Rind of ½ lemon, grated
½ pound fresh spinach,
   washed
2 tablespoons unsalted
   butter
2 egg whites, beaten

1 cup small-curd low-fat
   cottage cheese
⅓ cup grated lite
   Parmesan cheese
6 tablespoons low-fat milk
⅛ teaspoon ground black
   pepper
¼ teaspoon grated nutmeg

Preheat oven to 375°F. Add the lemon rind to the pie dough
and line the pan. Bake for 10 minutes (it will be partially
cooked). While pie shell bakes, briefly boil the spinach until
it is wilted. Drain the spinach, chop, add the butter, and mix.
In a separate bowl, beat the eggs, then mix in the cottage
cheese, Parmesan, milk, pepper, and nutmeg. Stir in the
spinach-and-butter mixture. Spread the resulting mixture in
the pie shell and bake for another 30 minutes, or until the pie
is browned and firm to the touch.

## Day Four

Breakfast
Fresh grapefruit half
Oatmeal Pancakes
Regular or herbal tea

Lunch
Fruit juice of choice
Water-packed tuna mixed with a spoonful of light mayonnaise, to which chopped onion, celery and dill have been added, served in a pita
Fruit of choice

Dinner
Fresh salad: lettuce, chopped carrots, tomatoes, radishes, cucumber, and low-fat/no-fat dressing
Spaghetti with turkey meatballs and lite Parmesan cheese
Low-fat yogurt, 1 bowl, with fresh fruit slices and almonds

## Oatmeal Pancakes

| | |
|---|---|
| 1 cup oat flakes or rolled oats | 2 tablespoons honey |
| 2 cups low-fat milk | 2 eggs, beaten |
| 1½ cups whole-grain flour | ¼ cup margarine |
| 1 teaspoon baking powder | Honey or low-calorie syrup |

Soak the oat flakes in milk overnight (if you use commercial rolled oats, soaking is unnecessary). Mix the flour, baking powder, and honey into the oat-and-milk mixture. Add the eggs and margarine. Spoon out small pancakes onto a lightly greased griddle, at medium-high heat, cooking pancakes on one side until bubbly, then turning them. Try to turn each pancake only once. Serve covered with honey or low-calorie syrup.

**Day Five**

Breakfast
Fruit juice of choice
English muffin with low-fat cream cheese
Nova Scotia salmon, 2 slices
Regular or herbal tea

Lunch
Large mixed fresh fruit salad: apples, pears, bananas,
    berries, etc.
Low-fat cottage cheese, 1 scoop
Whole grain bread, 2 slices, with low-fat spread

Dinner
Pineapple Chicken
Water chestnuts
Rice
Whole grain bread, 2 slices, with low-fat spread
Apple Baked in Honey

## Pineapple Chicken

1 clove garlic
¼ cup pineapple chunks
½ cup pineapple juice
¼ teaspoon powdered thyme

½ cup chicken broth
Ground black pepper
3 pounds assorted chicken
    parts

Combine the first six ingredients, add the chicken parts, and marinate for two hours in the refrigerator. Place the mixture in a skillet and heat until it boils, then cover and simmer for 45 minutes. Serve on a bed of rice.

## Apple Baked in Honey

4 large apples
½ cup water
1 teaspoon grated lemon rind

⅓ cup honey
Powdered cinnamon

Preheat oven to 475°F. Core the apples and place them in a baking dish. Combine the water, lemon rind, and honey. Pour this mixture over the apples, cover, and bake for 45 minutes, or until the apples are a tender golden brown (baste with the sauce several times during cooking). Serve with cinnamon to taste.

## Day Six

Breakfast
Fruit juice of choice
Egg White Omelet
Whole grain toast, 2 slices, with low-fat spread of choice
Regular or herbal tea

Lunch
Low-salt vegetable juice of choice
Hero sandwich on seven-grain bread: avocado slices, tomato slices, sprouts, lettuce, and low-fat mayonnaise (low-fat cheese slice optional)
Fruit of choice

Dinner
Tossed salad with low-fat dressing
Baked bluefish
Steamed broccoli
Baked potato
Whole grain roll with low-fat spread
Low-fat cookies with milk

Snack
Trail mix: shredded wheat, raisins, almond slivers, and small unsalted pretzels

## Egg White Omelet

| | |
|---|---|
| 3 egg whites | Scallions, chopped |
| 2 tablespoons water | ½ tomato, finely chopped |
| Ground black pepper | Nonfat cheddar cheese |
| Salt substitute | Chives |
| 1 tablespoon margarine | Parsley |

Preheat a skillet or omelet pan. Combine the egg whites, water, pepper, and a sprinkle of salt substitute. Beat for several minutes until the mixture is frothy. Melt the margarine in the pan, then add the egg white mixture. When the omelette is almost cooked, add the scallions, tomato, and cheese. Serve with a chive and parsley garnish.

**Day Seven**

Breakfast
Fruit juice of choice
Oatmeal with sliced bananas, almond slivers, and low-fat milk
Whole grain toast, 2 slices, with low-fat spread of choice
Regular or herbal tea

Lunch
Fresh Cabbage and Tomato Salad
Whole grain bread, 1 slice, with low-fat spread of choice
Fruit of choice

Dinner
Mixed green salad
Couscous with Shrimp
Sautéd snow peas
Whole grain bread, 1 slice
Low-fat/no-fat chocolate cake, 1 slice

Snacks
Healthy Cookies

## Healthy Cookies

2½ cups flour
½ teaspoon baking soda
⅓ cup olive oil

2 egg whites
¼ cup sugar
½ teaspoon vanilla

Preheat the oven to 375°F. Sift together the flour and baking soda. Cream the oil, egg whites, sugar, and vanilla. Combine the flour mixture and the creamed mixture. Press the dough out onto an unoiled nonstick baking sheet, making each cookie about ¼-inch thick. Bake for 15 minutes, or until lightly browned.

## Fresh Cabbage and Tomato Salad

1 head cabbage, sliced thin
2 tomatoes, cubed
1 cup radishes, sliced
2 teaspoons olive oil
¼ teaspoon ground
　black pepper

⅛ teaspoon salt
2 tablespoons rice wine
　vinegar (or lemon juice)
¼ teaspoon cayenne pepper
2 tablespoons chopped
　cilantro

Combine the cabbage, tomatoes, and radishes in a bowl. In another bowl, mix the remaining ingredients, and then pour this dressing over the vegetables.

**Day Eight**

Breakfast
Orange juice
Cottage Cheese Pineapple Surprise
Regular or herbal tea

Lunch
Fresh celery and carrot sticks
Bagel Pizza
Fruit of choice
Low-fat milk, 1 glass

Dinner
Turkey patties
Peas and cauliflower mix
Mashed potatoes
Whole grain roll
Low-fat ice cream

## Cottage Cheese Pineapple Surprise

½ cup low-fat cottage
   cheese
Chopped walnuts and
   almonds
¼ cup raisins

¼ cup pineapple cubes
¼ cup chopped dates
½ cantaloupe
Cinnamon

Combine the cottage cheese, nuts, raisins, pineapple cubes, and dates. Place this mixture in the half cantaloupe and broil for 2 minutes. Sprinkle with cinnamon just before serving.

## Bagel Pizza

1 whole grain bagel
2 tablespoons tomato sauce
1 ounce skim mozzarella
   cheese
2 tablespoons chopped,
   pitted black olives

Garlic powder, to taste
1 tablespoon grated
   Parmesan cheese

Cut the bagel in half and spread the tomato sauce on both halves. Slice the mozzarella, place it on the bagel halves, and top with the chopped olives. Sprinkle the halves with garlic powder and Parmesan cheese, then place them in the broiler and broil for two or three minutes.

## Day Nine

Breakfast
Grapefruit half
Granola with raisins and banana and apple slices
Regular or herbal tea

Lunch
Fresh vegetable salad
2 turkey or chicken hot dogs on buns
Homemade coleslaw (don't add salt)
Homemade potato salad (use lite mayonnaise)
Fruit of choice

Dinner
Turkey Meat Loaf
Mashed potatoes
Corn
Whole grain bread, 2 slices
Low-fat yogurt, 1 bowl, with fruit slice topping

Snack
Rice cakes with low-salt peanut butter

## Turkey Meat Loaf

| | |
|---|---|
| 1 pound ground turkey | 1 celery stalk |
| ⅓ cup skim milk | ½ teaspoon oregano |
| 1 egg white | ½ teaspoon basil |
| 2 slices whole grain bread | ½ teaspoon thyme |
| 1 small onion | 1 teaspoon mustard |
| 1 cup fresh parsley | Ground black pepper |

Preheat oven to 375°F. Place the ground turkey, milk, and egg white in a bowl and mix. Break or cut the bread into crumbs and add them to the turkey mixture. Chop the onion, parsley, and celery and sprinkle with oregano, basil, thyme, mustard, and pepper. Add the chopped vegetables to the turkey mixture and mix well. Form into a loaf, place in a baking dish, and bake for 45 minutes, or as long as it takes for meat loaf to become juicy and golden brown.

## Day Ten

Breakfast
Fruit juice of choice
Scrambled eggs, 2, sprinkled with pepper and chives
(no salt)
Whole grain bread, 2 slices, with jelly or jam
Regular or herbal tea

Lunch
Low-salt tomato juice
Tomatoes stuffed with tuna salad, 2
Low-fat cottage cheese, 1 scoop
Whole grain roll

Dinner
Fresh garden salad
Trout Vinaigrette
Rice topped with steamed vegetables
Whole grain bread, 1 slice
Choice of fresh fruit

Snack
Fresh pineapple chunks

## Trout Vinaigrette

¼ cup raisins
1 cup chicken broth
(or water)
4 tablespoons olive oil
⅓ cup chopped onion
1 clove garlic, minced
¼ cup finely chopped celery
½ teaspoon sage

½ teaspoon rosemary leaves
crushed
2 fresh trout, cleaned
¼ cup apple cider vinegar
1 teaspoon grated lemon peel
1 tablespoon unbleached
white flour
1 teaspoon unsalted butter

Soak the raisins in the broth. Warm the oil in a frying pan and sauté the onion, garlic, celery, sage, and rosemary until onion is transparent. Place the fish directly on top of the sauté and sprinkle it with the vinegar and lemon peel. Add the raisins and broth. Cover the pan and simmer over low heat for 10 minutes, or until the fish flakes when probed with a fork. Remove the fish from the pan, place on a serving dish, and lift off the top skin, up to the head. Blend the flour and butter with a fork, then stir it into the sauce in the frying pan and let it simmer and thicken while you stir. Pour the sauce over the fish and serve.

**Day Eleven**

Breakfast
Oatmeal with banana, raisins, and sunflower seeds
Whole grain bread, 2 slices
Regular or herbal tea

Lunch
Gazpacho
Steamed Corn Bread
Fresh black olives
Fruit of choice

Dinner
Appetizer of fresh snow peas
Roast chicken
Baked potato
Fresh lima beans
Whole grain bread sticks
Baked apple

## Gazpacho

¼ cup chopped scallions
½ cup chopped carrots
½ cup chopped cucumbers
½ cup chopped celery
½ cup chopped green
  peppers
¼ cup chopped radishes

2 cloves garlic, chopped
¼ cup olive oil
2 tablespoons vinegar
Large can low-salt tomato
  juice

Place the chopped scallions, carrots, cucumbers, celery, peppers, and radishes in a mixing bowl. Stir, then add the garlic. Add the oil to the vinegar, beating vigorously with a fork to make a vinaigrette, and add to the chopped vegetables. Stir, then slowly add the tomato juice. Store the mixture in refrigerator for at least 2 hours before serving. (Gazpacho is best if allowed to sit a day before serving.) Serve cold.

## Steamed Corn Bread

1 teaspoon baking powder
¼ teaspoon salt
4 tablespoons honey
2½ cups low-fat milk

4 cups cornmeal
¾ cup rice flour
4 egg whites
1 tablespoon olive oil

Preheat oven to 250°F. Combine the baking powder, salt, honey, and milk in a bowl. Stir until the dry ingredients have dissolved. Slowly mix in the cornmeal and rice flour, stirring until batter comes to an even consistency. Beat one egg white for 30 seconds, then add to mixture with oil. Beat the 3 remaining egg whites, then add to mixture. Fold in the oil and beat some more. Place the batter in a piepan and bake for 20 to 30 minutes, or until corn bread has a pleasant crust.

## Day Twelve

Breakfast
Fruit juice of choice
Hard-boiled egg
Whole grain bread, 2 slices
Regular or herbal tea

Lunch
Large fruit salad: apple, banana, cantaloupe slices, straw-
berries, and almonds
Low-fat cottage cheese, a small serving, with sunflower
seeds
Whole grain bread, 1 slice

Dinner
Bean salad: mixed precooked black beans, white beans,
chickpeas, and tofu chunks, topped with sprinkle of
sesame oil and sesame seeds
Cauliflower-Carrot Delight
Rice
Low-fat cookies

Snack
Celery and carrot sticks with a low-fat dip

## Cauliflower-Carrot Delight

1 cauliflower
5 carrots
½ teaspoon honey
2 teaspoons olive oil

1½ tablespoons whole grain
   flour
2 cups low-fat milk
Nutmeg

Steam the cauliflower until it's tender. Cook the carrots until they are pulpy, then puree and add the honey. Mix oil, flour and milk, add carrots, and cook the mixture over medium heat, stirring continually until it is well thickened. Pour the carrot sauce over the cauliflower, add a pinch of nutmeg, and serve.

## Day Thirteen

Breakfast
Fruit juice of choice
Bagel or black bread spread with low-fat cream cheese
Nova Scotia salmon, 2 slices (put on bread or bagel)
Regular or herbal tea

Lunch
Coleslaw with carrots and raisins
Pureed tofu with a dash of curry powder, spread on:
Whole grain bread, 2 slices
Applesauce with sprinkle of cinnamon

Dinner
Marinated Green Bean Salad
Cooked bulgur
Sautéed vegetables with chicken slices
Fresh garden salad
Fruit Compote

## Marinated Green Bean Salad

1 onion, chopped
¼ cup olive oil
2 tomatoes, peeled, sliced

½ cup water
1 pound fresh whole green
  beans

Sauté the onion in the oil for several minutes, then add tomatoes, water, and green beans. Cook until the green beans become tender. Place in a bowl and refrigerate for a day. Serve cold.

## Fruit Compote

¾ cup water
½ cup sugar
2 teaspoons lemon juice
1 piece lemon peel
½ teaspoon vanilla extract
2 mangoes, sliced

1 pineapple, sliced
3 bananas, cut into diagonal
  pieces
Mint leaves, fresh (optional)
Nonfat sour cream

Combine the water with the sugar, lemon juice, lemon peel, and vanilla extract in a saucepan. Bring to a boil, then reduce the heat and add the fruit. Cook at a low heat for 5 minutes. Pour the syrup into a cup. Remove the lemon peel and refrigerate the fruit for 2 hours. Arrange the fruit in a serving dish and pour 3 teaspoonfuls of syrup over it. Add the mint leaves and serve with nonfat sour cream.

**Day Fourteen**

Breakfast
Fruit juice of choice
Cereal with apple and banana slices and almonds
Whole grain bread, 1 slice, with low-fat spread of choice
Regular or herbal tea

Lunch
Fruit or vegetable juice of choice
Small garden salad: carrots, celery, and tomatoes, with
    low-fat dressing
Chicken salad sandwich on whole grain bread
Fruit of choice

Dinner
Fresh salad
Chicken Creole
Corn
Mashed potatoes
Low-fat yogurt topped with fruit slices

Snack
Low-salt, unbuttered popcorn

## Chicken Creole

1 pound boneless, skinless
  chicken
½ teaspoon paprika
1 green pepper, sliced
1 cup chopped fresh
  mushrooms
1 cup low-salt whole
  tomatoes

½ cup chopped celery
1 large onion, sliced
½ cup water
Cayenne pepper
2 tablespoons chopped
  parsley

Slice the chicken, sprinkle with the paprika, and brown in a skillet. Remove the chicken from skillet and add green peppers, mushrooms, tomatoes, celery, onion, and water. Bring the mixture to a boil and simmer for 10 minutes. Return the chicken to the skillet, add a pinch of cayenne pepper (to taste), and allow the chicken and vegetable mixture to simmer for 30 to 40 minutes, or until done. Garnish with the parsley and serve.

## Day Fifteen

Breakfast
Fruit juice of choice
Bran cereal with raisin, almond, and banana topping
Low-fat milk
Regular or herbal tea

Lunch
Spinach salad with low-fat dressing
Whole grain bread, 2 slices, with low-fat spread
Fruit of choice

Dinner
Bean and Pasta Soup
Large fresh vegetable salad
Garlic bread
Fresh pears in syrup

Snack
Honeydew slices
Whole grain roll

## Bean and Pasta Soup

½ cup elbow or shell
macaroni
2 tablespoons canola oil
1 clove garlic, minced
1 onion, chopped
1 green pepper, chopped
1 6-ounce can tomato paste
3 cups stock or water

1¾ cups canned kidney
beans
1½ cups canned chickpeas
½ teaspoon savory
½ teaspoon thyme
Cayenne pepper, to taste
Fresh ground black pepper
Grated Parmesan

Cook the pasta. While the pasta is cooking, heat the oil in a saucepan. Stir in the garlic, onion, and green pepper and sauté till brown. Add the remaining ingredients to the saucepan. Cover and cook for 10 to 15 minutes. When the sauce is done, pour it over the pasta. Serve with fresh ground black pepper and grated Parmesan.

## Day Sixteen

**Breakfast**
Fruit juice of choice
Oatmeal with raisins, almonds, and banana slices
Regular or herbal tea

**Lunch**
Fruit or vegetable juice of choice
Chicken salad sandwich with sprouts and tomatoes on whole grain roll
Low-fat cottage cheese, 1 scoop
Fruit of choice

**Dinner**
Fresh salad
Spicy Baked Fish
Steamed brussels sprouts
Baked potato
Fresh strawberries in low-fat milk

**Snack**
Tofu slices with lite soy sauce, grated ginger, and sesame seeds

## Spicy Baked Fish

1 tablespoon safflower oil
½ cup chopped onion
3 cloves garlic
  (medium-sized)
1 egg white
Chili powder, to taste
1 16-ounce can skinless
  tomatoes, chopped

1 tablespoon skim milk
4 flounder fillets
½ cup cornmeal
½ cup shredded low-fat
  mozzarella
Ground black pepper, to taste

Preheat oven to 350°F. Heat the oil in a saucepan and sauté the onions and garlic until browned. Add the chili powder, and tomatoes. Stir mixture while cooking over high heat for several minutes, then simmer for 15 minutes, stirring occasionally. In a shallow dish, beat the egg white and skim milk together. Dip the flounder fillets in this egg mixture, then coat with cornmeal. Place the fillets in a baking dish and pour the tomato sauce over them. Add the shredded mozzarella and pepper, and bake for 20 to 30 minutes, or until the fish begins to flake.

**Day Seventeen**

Breakfast
Fruit juice of choice
Scrambled eggs, 2
Bran muffin with low-fat spread
Regular or herbal tea

Lunch
2 fresh celery stalks
Sprout and Fruit Salad
Whole grain bread, 1 slice, with low-fat spread
Fruit of choice

Dinner
Fresh garden salad
Baked halibut
Artichoke with olive oil
Whole grain bread, 1 slice
Low-fat ice cream

Snack
Slices of fresh cucumber with nonfat yogurt
Sunflower and raisin mix

## Sprout and Fruit Salad

1 cup bean sprouts
½ cup fresh orange slices
2 stalks celery, diced
½ cup water chestnuts
¼ cup hulled walnuts

½ cup sliced pineapple bits
¼ cup low-fat yogurt
1 teaspoon honey
1 teaspoon curry powder
½ teaspoon fresh grated
ginger

Mix the sprouts, orange slices, celery, water chestnuts, walnuts, and pineapple bits in a bowl. To make the dressing, mix the yogurt, honey, curry powder, and grated ginger in a separate bowl. Pour the dressing over the salad and serve.

## Day Eighteen

Breakfast
Fruit juice of choice
Whole grain blueberry pancakes
Choice of syrup or no-fat sour cream topping
Regular or herbal tea

Lunch
Fruit or vegetable juice of choice
Fresh avocado half sprinkled with lemon juice
Low-fat cottage cheese, 1 scoop
Whole grain bread, 2 slices
Fresh fruit of choice

Dinner
Tomato and onion slices
Welsh Rarebit on toast
Date-Nut Tarts

## Welsh Rarebit

3 tablespoons olive oil
1 pound low-fat cheddar
   cheese, cubed
½ cup nonalcoholic beer

⅛ teaspoon cayenne pepper
¼ teaspoon dry mustard
1 egg, beaten
Ground pepper, to taste

Heat the oil in the top of a double boiler. Add the cheddar cubes and cook until just melted. Add the beer slowly, then the spices, then the egg. Cook for several minutes more and serve hot over whole grain toast. Add pepper, if desired.

## Date-Nut Tarts

Pastry for double-crust pie
2 egg whites
½ cup honey
½ cup pecans or walnuts

½ cup finely chopped dates
1 teaspoon vanilla
¼ cup olive oil

Preheat oven to 350°F. Roll out the dough on a floured board and cut it into 4-inch circles (a 4-inch circle of dough will fit into muffin-tin cups 1¼ inches in diameter). Press these into muffin-tin cups. Beat the egg whites, then add the honey and stir vigorously. Stir in the nuts, dates, vanilla, and oil. Fill each pastry cup about one-quarter full. Bake 25 minutes, or until browned with a firm center.

**Day Nineteen**

Breakfast
Fruit juice of choice
Whole grain cereal with banana and apple slices and almonds
Whole grain bread, 1 slice, with low-fat spread
Regular or herbal tea

Lunch
Fruit juice of choice
Tomato, cucumber, and bean curd slices
2 turkey burgers on whole grain rolls

Dinner
Cucumber-Yogurt Soup
Lamb chops
Peas
Whole grain bread, 1 slice
Low-fat cake of choice

## Cucumber-Yogurt Soup

2 cucumbers
1 pint low-fat yogurt
¼ teaspoon ground cumin
Worcestershire sauce

2 tablespoons chopped
   fresh dill
Ground black pepper, to taste

Peel the cucumbers and run them through a blender till pulped, and pour into a bowl. Add the yogurt, the cumin, and a dash of Worcestershire. Mix well and refrigerate for several hours. Sprinkle the dill and pepper on top and serve.

**Day Twenty**

Breakfast
Fruit juice of choice
Low-fat cheese omelet
Whole grain bread, 2 slices
Regular or herbal tea

Lunch
Fruit or vegetable juice of choice
Crudités: sliced carrots, radish, celery, and cucumber,
with low-fat dip
Low-fat mozzarella cheese, 2 slices
Fruit of choice

Dinner
Low-fat yogurt with minced garlic cloves and fresh car-
rot and cucumber slices mixed in
Indian-Style Lamb
Rice
Chutney
Indian chapati, or 1 slice whole grain bread
Mixed fruit: grapes, sliced fresh orange, cantaloupe,
and banana

Snack
Rice crackers spread with jelly and unsalted peanut
butter

## Indian-Style Lamb

4 medium-sized onions,
  chopped
3 cloves garlic, chopped
2 tablespoons canola oil
1½ teaspoons curry powder
  or garam masala

1 tablespoon chopped fresh
  ginger
1½ teaspoon turmeric
2 pounds boneless stewing
  lamb
2 cups low-fat yogurt

Sauté the onions and garlic in the oil for 3 minutes. Then add the curry powder or garam masala, ginger, and turmeric and cook for several minutes. Add the lamb and cook until mixture is brown. Add the yogurt, cover, and simmer slowly for 1 hour, or until the lamb is tender. Serve with rice and chutney.

## Day Twenty-one

Breakfast
Grapefruit half
Shredded wheat with low-fat milk
Whole grain bread, 1 slice
Regular or herbal tea

Lunch
Fruit or vegetable juice of choice
Tuna fish sandwich on whole wheat bread (use water-packed tuna)
Low-fat cheese, 1 slice
Fruit of choice

Dinner
Garden salad
Asparagus Quiche
Broccoli
Whole grain roll with low-fat spread
Fruit of choice

## Asparagus Quiche

*For the crust:*

½ cup all-purpose flour
⅝ cup whole wheat flour
¼ teaspoon sugar

¼ teaspoon salt
3½ ounces skim milk
¼ cup olive oil

*For the filling:*

¾ cup low-fat grated Swiss
  cheese
2 cups asparagus
¼ cup scallions
2 teaspoons minced red
  pepper

3 egg whites
¾ cup evaporated skim milk
½ teaspoon white pepper
½ cup nonfat yogurt
½ teaspoon salt

Preheat oven to 450°F. Mix the flours, sugar, and salt in a bowl. Add the milk and oil. Stir with a fork until well mixed, then form into a small ball. Roll out the dough between two 12-inch squares of waxed paper. Peel off the top square, invert the piecrust, and place it on a 9-inch piepan. Carefully peel off the paper and gently fit the piecrust into the piepan. Flute the edges and prick the pastry with a fork. Bake for 5 to 7 minutes. Remove from oven.

Sprinkle ¼ cup of the Swiss cheese over the crust. Layer the asparagus, scallions, minced red pepper, and the remaining ½ cup of the Swiss cheese. Blend the egg whites, evaporated milk, white pepper, yogurt, and salt and pour over the asparagus mixture in the piecrust. Return the filled crust to the oven and bake for 10 minutes at 450°F. Reduce heat to 325°F. and bake for another 20 to 25 minutes, or until a knife inserted in the center of the quiche comes out clean. Let stand 5 to 10 minutes before serving.

## Day Twenty-two

Breakfast
Fruit juice of choice
Hard-boiled egg
Whole grain bread, 2 slices, with low-fat spread of
    choice
Regular or herbal tea

Lunch
Fruit or vegetable juice of choice
Sliced tomatoes sprinkled with basil (fresh basil, if pos-
    sible)
Eggplant with Sesame Seed Sandwich
Fruit of choice

Dinner
Garden salad
Roast chicken
Fresh string beans
Baked potato
Whole grain roll with low-fat spread
No-fat frozen yogurt

Snack
Orange-Pineapple Slush

## Eggplant with Sesame Seed Sandwich

2 eggplants
⅛ teaspoon sesame seeds

Balsamic vinegar
Whole grain bread

Remove the skin from the eggplants. Cut the eggplants into thin slices and roast the slices on a grill. Roast the sesame seeds separately in a skillet over a low flame or in a toaster oven. Sprinkle the sesame seeds on the roasted eggplant. Sprinkle balsamic vinegar on the bread and add the eggplant as a sandwich filling.

## Orange-Pineapple Slush

4 ounces concentrated
frozen orange juice
3 ounces crushed frozen
pineapple

1 tablespoon vanilla extract
1 cup skim milk
½ cup water
1 cup ice cubes

Blend all ingredients in a blender and serve immediately.

## Day Twenty-three

Breakfast
Fruit juice of choice
Whole grain cereal with bananas and raisins
Whole grain bread, 1 slice
Regular or herbal tea

Lunch
Fruit or vegetable juice of choice
Deli spread: low-fat lunch meat, sliced tomatoes, carrots, cucumber slices, low-fat cheese, radishes, cauliflower flowerets, sprouts
Whole grain bread, 2 slices, with low-fat spread of choice
Fruit of choice

Dinner
Garden salad
Tofu Chili
Low-fat yogurt
Whole grain crackers
Fruit of choice

## Tofu Chili

2 packages firm tofu
  (bean curd)
1 large onion, diced
½ teaspoon grated fresh
  ginger
½ diced green pepper
2 cloves garlic, minced
1 teaspoon oil

4 ounces tomato sauce
4 cups cooked kidney beans
¼ teaspoon salt
Chili powder to taste
¼ teaspoon black pepper
4 teaspoons vinegar
3 cups diced fresh tomatoes

Crumble the tofu into a bowl. In a large pot, sauté the onion, ginger, green pepper, and garlic in a teaspoonful of oil until onions are tender. Add the tofu and sauté 5 minutes longer. Mix the rest of the ingredients and simmer for ½ hour, stirring frequently. Serve with no-fat yogurt and crackers.

## Day Twenty-four

Breakfast
Fruit juice of choice
Low-fat cheese melted on 2 slices of whole wheat bread
Regular or herbal tea

Lunch
Fruit or vegetable juice of choice
Chicken salad sandwich with lettuce and tomato on
    whole grain bread
Low-fat cottage cheese, 1 scoop
Fruit of choice

Dinner
Garden salad
Grilled Tofu Masala
Steamed broccoli
Steamed spinach
Whole grain bread, 1 slice
Rice Pudding

## Grilled Tofu Masala

10 slices firm tofu
3 teaspoons lemon juice
1 teaspoon garlic powder
½ cup fresh coriander
  (cilantro), finely chopped

3 teaspoons grated ginger
Salt and pepper to taste

Preheat oven to 375°F. Marinate the tofu in the lemon juice with the garlic powder added for one hour in the refrigerator. Grill the tofu slices 7 minutes on each side. Make a hole in the side of each tofu slice for stuffing. Stuff the slices with the coriander, ginger, salt, and pepper, transfer to a baking dish, and bake at 375°F. for 10 minutes. Serve with vegetables.

## Rice Pudding

6 cups water
2 cinnamon sticks
1 cup rice
3 cups skim milk

⅔ cup sugar
⅛ teaspoon salt
Ground cinnamon

Place the water and cinnamon sticks in a medium saucepan and bring to a boil. Stir in the rice and cook over low heat for 30 minutes, or until the rice is soft and all the water has evaporated from the pan. Add skim milk, sugar, and salt. Cook for another 15 minutes, or until the mixture has thickened. Serve sprinkled with cinnamon.

## Day Twenty-five

Breakfast
Fruit juice of choice
Oatmeal with sliced banana and low-fat milk
Whole grain toast, 2 slices, with jelly or jam
Regular or herbal tea

Lunch
Large mixed fruit salad: apples, pears, bananas, berries, etc.
Low-fat cottage cheese, 1 scoop
Whole grain bread, 2 slices, with low-fat spread

Dinner
Mexican Pozole Soup
Carrot slices, onion, garlic, and bean curd sautéed in olive oil
Rice (serve vegetables over rice and sprinkle with sesame seeds)
Whole grain bread, 1 slice
Low-fat ice cream

## Mexican Pozole Soup

1 tablespoon olive oil
2 pounds chicken, cubed
1 onion, chopped
1 clove garlic, chopped
⅛ teaspoon salt
⅛ teaspoon pepper

¼ cup cilantro
1 15-ounce can stewed
  tomatoes
2 ounces tomato paste
1 can hominy

Heat the oil in a large pot. Sauté the chicken. Add the onion, garlic, salt, pepper, cilantro, and enough water to cover the chicken. Cover the pot and cook over low heat until the chicken is tender. Add the tomatoes and tomato paste. Continue cooking for about 20 minutes. Add the hominy and continue cooking for another 15 minutes over a low flame, stirring occasionally. If the soup is too thick, add water for desired consistency.

## Day Twenty-six

Breakfast
Fruit juice of choice
Fresh apple slices on granola cereal
Regular or herbal tea

Lunch
Fruit or vegetable juice of choice
Sliced carrot and celery sticks
Fresh-ground peanut butter with jelly on whole wheat bread
Fruit of choice

Dinner
Marinated Green Bean Salad (see recipe, Day Thirteen)
Cooked Bulgur
Sautéed vegetables and chicken slices (serve over bulgur)
Millet Dessert

## Cooked Bulgur

1 cup wheat berries            ⅛ teaspoon salt
2 cups water

Preheat oven to 300°F. Boil wheat berries in the water for 1 hour, adding the salt in the last 15 minutes. Strain off the water and bake the kernels at 300°F for 45 minutes to 1 hour, or until all moisture has evaporated. Allow the grain to cool, then grind it to a coarse consistency in a blender or food processor.

## Millet Dessert

2 cups milk             1 orange
¼ cup honey          2 egg whites
¼ cup cracked millet    ½ teaspoon vanilla extract
1 lemon

Warm the milk. Dissolve the honey in the milk, then add the millet. Boil for 30 to 45 minutes, or until the grain is soft and porridgelike, stirring frequently. Extract juice from the lemon and orange. Add the egg whites to the millet, stirring well, then place the mixture on stove and simmer for several minutes. Remove, add the vanilla and the lemon and orange juice, and stir. Chill before serving.

## Day Twenty-seven

Breakfast
Fruit juice of choice
Stewed prunes
Cream of Wheat with low-fat milk and sliced banana
Regular or herbal tea

Lunch
Fruit or vegetable juice of choice
Turkey burger on bun
Unsalted chips or crackers
Low-fat cottage cheese, 1 scoop
Fruit of choice

Dinner
Garden salad
Squash Bisque
Broiled bluefish
Baked potato
Whole grain bread, 1 slice
Fruit of choice

## Squash Bisque

2 teaspoons olive oil
1 cup chopped onion
½ cup chopped apple
4 cups butternut squash, peeled and cubed
4 cups chicken stock

1 teaspoon salt
¼ teaspoon ground black pepper
1 teaspoon dried chervil
¼ teaspoon ground nutmeg
¼ cup evaporated skim milk

In a large, heavy saucepan, heat the oil. Add the onion and sauté until soft. Add the chopped apple, butternut squash, chicken stock, salt, pepper, chervil, and nutmeg. Cover and simmer for 15 to 20 minutes. Allow the mixture to cool. Pour into an electric blender or food processor and puree until smooth. Return the purée to the saucepan and bring to a simmer. Stir in the evaporated milk and continue cooking until mixture is heated through. Optional: When serving, garnish with 1 teaspoonful of mixed chopped hazelnuts and walnuts.

## Day Twenty-eight

Breakfast
Fruit juice of choice
Hard-boiled egg
Whole grain bread, 2 slices
Regular or herbal tea

Lunch
Fruit or vegetable juice of choice
Hot Dog Pizza
Fruit of choice

Dinner
Garden salad
Bean Tikki
Steamed mixed vegetables: carrots, peas, turnips
Whole grain bread, 1 slice, with low-fat spread
Low-fat yogurt with fruit

## Hot Dog Pizza

½ cup chopped onion
2 tablespoons oil
1 can vegetarian baked
   beans
Pita bread buns

3 chicken hot dogs, sliced
   into bite-sized pieces
½ ounce low-fat cheddar,
   shredded

Preheat oven to 375°F. Sauté the onion with oil in skillet until tender. Mix in the beans, cover, and cook 3 or 4 minutes. Place the pita on a baking sheet, top with hot dog slices, cheese, and onion-bean mixture. Bake for several minutes, or until the pita is crispy and the cheese melted.

## Bean Tikki

8 ounces tofu
½ teaspoon ground black
   pepper
2 tablespoons chopped
   onion
¼ teaspoon salt

4 teaspoons chopped celery
4 tablespoons shredded
   carrot
4 teaspoons bread crumbs
Pam cooking oil spray

Preheat oven to 350°F. Mash the tofu in a bowl. Mix in all the other ingredients except the bread crumbs and the Pam. Shape the mixture into into 8 patties. Sprinkle ½ teaspoonful of the bread crumbs on each side of the patties. Spray a baking pan with Pam for 3 seconds, then bake until the patties are crisp and brown. Serve with chopped fresh coriander, chutney, or salsa, if desired.

## Day Twenty-nine

Breakfast
Fruit juice of choice
Low-fat yogurt with banana slices
Regular or herbal tea

Lunch
Fruit or vegetable juice of choice
Tabouli
Whole grain bread, 1 slice, with low-fat spread
Fruit of choice

Dinner
Garden salad
Roast lamb
Baked potato
Lima beans
Healthy Chocolate Cake

## Tabouli

¾ cup bulgur (cracked wheat)
1 cup boiling water
3 tomatoes, chopped
1½ cups finely chopped
  parsley
½ cup finely chopped
  fresh mint

2 cloves garlic, chopped
½ teaspoon ground black
  pepper
¼ teaspoon salt
½ cup lemon juice
½ cup olive oil

Cover the bulgur with the hot water and let stand for 1 hour. Mix in the chopped ingredients, then add the pepper, salt, lemon juice, and olive oil. Mix thoroughly, refrigerate for an hour or so, and serve with slices of low-fat cheese, olives, and whole grain bread.

## Healthy Chocolate Cake

2¼ cups flour
1 cup sugar
1 ounce unsweetened cocoa
1 teaspoon baking soda
½ teaspoon salt

½ cup plus 1 tablespoon
  olive oil
1¼ cups skim milk
4 egg whites

Preheat oven to 350°F. Grease a 13 x 9-inch baking pan and line the bottom with waxed paper. Sift the flour, sugar, cocoa, baking soda, and salt into bowl of an electric beater. Add the remaining ingredients. Beat at low speed until the dry ingredients are moistened, then beat 2 minutes at medium speed. Pour the batter into the prepared pan. Bake 30 to 40 minutes, or until you can stick a toothpick in the center of the cake and bring it out clean.

## Day Thirty

Breakfast
Fruit juice of choice
Oatmeal with sliced banana and low-fat milk
Regular or herbal tea

Lunch
Fruit juice of choice
Crudités: sliced celery, carrots, cucumber, and radish
Corn Bread and Black Bean Spread
Fruit of choice

Dinner
Garden salad
Roast chicken
Boiled carrots with dash of dill and olive oil
Baked potato
Whole grain bread, 1 slice, with low-fat spread
Healthy Chocolate Cake (see recipe, Day Twenty-nine)

# Corn Bread and Black Bean Spread

*The Corn Bread*

| | |
|---|---|
| 1 tsp. baking powder | 4 cups cornmeal |
| ¼ tablespoons salt | ¾ cup rice flour |
| 4 tablespoons honey | 4 egg whites |
| 2½ cups low-fat milk | 1 tablespoons olive oil |

Preheat oven to 300°F. Combine the baking powder, salt, honey, and milk in a bowl. Stir until dry ingredients are well dissolved. Slowly mix in the cornmeal and rice flour, stirring until the batter reaches an even consistency. Add 1 egg white to the batter along with the olive oil. Then add the three remaining whites, folding in oil and whites until they are evenly distributed. Pour batter into a piepan and bake for 20 or 30 minutes, or until the bread is done to a golden brown.

*The Black Bean Spread*

| | |
|---|---|
| 2 cups dried black beans | Dried basil, a pinch |
| 2 medium onions, diced | Ground black pepper, a pinch |
| 2 cloves garlic, chopped | ¼ teaspoon salt |
| Fresh dill, a pinch | Juice of 1 lemon |

Boil the black beans until they're tender. Combine the onions, garlic, dill, basil, pepper, and salt in a mixing bowl, then add the lemon juice. Stir, then add the beans and put the mixture into a blender. Blend until it is finely pureed. Serve on corn bread or whole wheat crackers.

## A Call to Action

There are several messages that we hope have come through clearly in the different sections of this book.

The first is that high blood pressure is both a common ailment and a potentially dangerous one. While millions of Americans suffer from this insidious disease, a large percent of sufferers pay it no attention, thinking—quite erroneously—that it will go away on its own. Others are simply unaware that they have the disease, or that it is harmful. And since hypertension rarely produces symptoms, a person with high blood pressure can go for decades blithely insensible to the risks.

But be assured: Those who follow this course put themselves at risk. For as far as the "silent killer" goes, a head-in-the-sand approach can produce a number of serious physical ailments, including heart disease, kidney failure, and stroke.

The second message that anyone concerned with hypertension is well advised to heed is that while high blood pressure is potentially hazardous to your health, it is also eminently treatable. Whatever preventive or curative modalities you may choose, *do* treat this condition. There is no downside to treatment, and a lot of up.

Finally, we hope it has been made clear in these pages that high blood pressure is a disease of both organic and external origins—that it originates from genetic and biological factors, yes, but also from the environmental influences that affect us every day of our lives at home and at work.

Throughout this book we have discussed these influences and reviewed methods for turning risk factors into allies. Undue stress, improper diet, lack of exercise, overuse of alcohol and tobacco, and all the rest take their toll. Conversely, stress reduction, daily exercise, careful diet, and temperate living make a real difference, not only in the way we feel but in the number of years we live.

For people who suffer from hypertension, therefore, lifestyle changes are often all that is required to keep blood pressure irregularities in check. Sometimes just modifying one variable like diet or physical activity does the trick. And if these approaches don't solve the problem entirely, they still serve as powerful supplements to standard medications.

The efforts we make to improve our habits of living and to avoid proven menaces to cardiovascular health really do make a difference, sometimes a profound difference. All we need do is take advantage of the many lifestyle tools that are already at hand.

The choice is yours.

# The PDR® Family Guide to Over-the-Counter Drugs™

For the first time, the most trusted name in medical publishing, *Physicians' Desk Reference®*, has produced a comprehensive, authoritative, and reliable consumer guide to over-the-counter drugs. Its features include

- The uses, active ingredients, proper dosages, and side effects of each medication

- Handy comparison tables to help you select the best product for each ailment

- Symptoms of vitamin deficiency—and the signs of overdose

- Special cautions for seniors, expectant mothers, and infants

- And much more!

Published by Ballantine Books.
Available wherever books are sold.

# The PDR® Family Guide Encyclopedia of Medical Care™

Now the most trusted name in medical publishing—the source physicians and pharmacists turn to—puts expert guidance and information at your fingertips. With a comprehensive alphabetical listing of common and unusual ailments that afflict both children and adults—plus a unique index that matches your signs and symptoms to possible conditions—this is a reassuring home health care reference. Inside you'll find

- Detailed instructions for home care

- Possible causes of ailments

- When to call your doctor for further care

- And much more

Published by Ballantine Books.
Available in bookstores everywhere.